The LifeWave Patch Therapy Bible

A practical guide on using phototherapy effectively for healing,boost energy,relieve pain and improve sleep

ISBN: 9798343893083
Johnathon Engle

TABLE OF CONTENT

INTRODUCTION

Overview of LifeWave Patch Therapy

Recently, more and more people have been drawn to non-invasive, natural treatments that tap into the body's own ability to heal itself. Among these new therapies, LifeWave Patch Therapy has captured interest for its unique approach to using light for healing. This method aims to boost energy, alleviate pain, and enhance sleep quality. This introduction aims to offer a comprehensive look at LifeWave Patch Therapy, exploring its scientific basis and the important role that light plays in enhancing our overall health and well-being.

What is LifeWave Patch Therapy?

LifeWave Patch Therapy is an innovative wellness approach that harnesses light to encourage the body's inherent healing abilities. Created by LifeWave, a company established in 2004 by David Schmidt, these patches aim to engage with particular acupressure points on the body, assisting in balancing energy flow, enhancing physical performance, and speeding up recovery. LifeWave patches stand apart from traditional patches by not relying on drugs or chemicals to penetrate the skin. They use a distinctive method that involves phototherapy, rather than a transdermal approach.

LifeWave Patch Therapy is fundamentally about applying small adhesive patches to specific spots on the skin. These patches contain unique organic materials that respond to body heat by reflecting certain wavelengths of light. The light that bounces off interacts with the skin and tissues, encouraging certain cellular activities to take place. The patches communicate with the body through light signals, encouraging it to engage its natural healing and regenerative processes.

The versatility of LifeWave patches is one of their key benefits. People use them for a range of health benefits, such as easing pain, boosting energy, enhancing sleep quality, detoxifying the body, and promoting a youthful appearance. Among the well-loved LifeWave patches, you'll find the X39 patch, known for its ability to encourage stem cell activation, aiding in tissue repair and regeneration; the Energy Enhancer patch, which helps to elevate vitality and endurance; and the IceWave patch, crafted specifically for alleviating pain.

One of the most attractive aspects of LifeWave Patch Therapy is how simple it is to use. The patches can be applied without any specialized medical training, making them easy to use for both healthcare professionals and anyone looking for natural solutions to common health issues. People can place the patches right on their skin, often at acupressure points, to address particular health issues. LifeWave patches are gaining traction among athletes, wellness seekers, and individuals exploring options beyond traditional medication treatments.

Understanding Phototherapy

To truly grasp how LifeWave Patch Therapy operates, it's essential to delve into the science behind phototherapy, also known as light therapy. For centuries, people have turned to phototherapy in different ways, starting with ancient civilizations that harnessed the healing power of sunlight, all the way to today's advanced methods like laser therapy and LED treatments. Phototherapy operates on a straightforward yet impactful principle: light has the ability to affect biological processes within our bodies at the cellular level, encouraging healing and regeneration.

Phototherapy involves using particular wavelengths of light to interact with the skin and deeper tissues, initiating a series of biochemical responses. When light reaches the skin, it can be taken in by cells, especially by special molecules called chromophores that are sensitive to light. These chromophores can be found in different cell structures, like mitochondria, which are often referred to as the powerhouses of the cell. When light shines on them, mitochondria can boost their production of adenosine triphosphate (ATP), which serves as the energy currency for the cell. This increase in cellular energy helps speed up repair and regeneration, resulting in quicker healing and better function.

Besides enhancing cellular energy, phototherapy can also affect the production of nitric oxide, a vital molecule that helps manage blood flow, decrease inflammation, and ease muscle tension. Phototherapy can help improve circulation, boost collagen production, alleviate pain, and activate the body's natural anti-inflammatory responses.

LifeWave patches utilize a type of light therapy called photobiomodulation. LifeWave patches stand out from traditional phototherapy devices because they harness the body's own infrared radiation instead of relying on external light sources. The patches are crafted using unique materials that bounce certain wavelengths of light back into the body, activating the same biochemical responses that traditional phototherapy achieves. The patches can function well on their own, without needing electricity or any outside light to help them out.

LifeWave patches stand out because they can address specific health issues by influencing various biological pathways. The X39 patch works by encouraging the production of stem cells, which helps the body heal damaged tissues and regenerate cells more effectively. The IceWave patch focuses on pain pathways, helping to reduce inflammation and offering quick relief from pain.

LifeWave patches operate using light and energy instead of chemicals or pharmaceuticals, making them non-invasive and nearly free of side effects. This provides a secure choice for people of all ages, including those with chronic health issues who might be looking for alternatives to medication-based treatments.

The Role of Light Therapy in Enhancing Health and Well-Being

Light plays an essential role in our lives. Our bodies have developed remarkable ways to engage with light, influencing everything from our sleep patterns to our immune health and energy levels. Studies indicate that light is essential for our health and overall well-being, and when we experience imbalances in light exposure, it can result in various health problems.

One of the most recognized effects of light is its role in regulating the body's internal clock, which influences sleep, metabolism, and hormone production. Being in natural light during the day helps our brains stay awake and engaged, while when night falls and light fades, our bodies start to produce melatonin, a hormone that encourages us to sleep. When our natural body clocks get thrown off, often due to excessive artificial light at night or not enough sunlight during the day, it can result in sleepless nights, tiredness, and even impact our mood, potentially leading to feelings of sadness or depression.

In addition to influencing sleep, light significantly impacts our energy levels and mood. Sunlight is a wonderful natural source of vitamin D, which plays a crucial role in keeping our bones healthy, supporting our immune system, and helping to regulate our mood. Low levels of vitamin D can be associated with feelings of tiredness, a less robust immune system, and even sadness. Light therapy has been utilized to help with seasonal affective disorder (SAD), a form of depression that tends to arise during the darker months when we have less natural light.

Alongside its impact on mood and sleep, light therapy has demonstrated notable advantages for managing pain. Studies indicate that light therapy may help lessen inflammation, support wound healing, and ease pain in conditions like arthritis, fibromyalgia, and chronic back pain. Phototherapy for pain relief is becoming more popular as it provides a natural option compared to conventional painkillers, which often come with undesirable side effects or the risk of dependence.

Light therapy also plays an important role in promoting youthful skin and overall skin health. Light therapy can help your skin by boosting collagen production and enhancing blood flow, which may lead to fewer wrinkles, better skin elasticity, and faster wound healing. This is often utilized in skin care treatments for issues such as acne, psoriasis, and eczema.

Considering the various ways light impacts our bodies, it's understandable that phototherapy has emerged as a vital component in contemporary wellness approaches. LifeWave Patch Therapy uses light to create a comprehensive approach to health, delivering advantages that go beyond just alleviating symptoms. LifeWave patches work by focusing on the body's natural energy systems, helping to heal from the inside out. They aim to tackle the underlying issues that cause imbalances, ultimately supporting a return to overall well-being.

LifeWave Patch Therapy brings together the timeless wisdom of light-based healing and modern technology, offering a gentle and effective way to boost health and well-being. By grasping the science behind phototherapy and recognizing the vital role of light in our well-being, people can fully harness the benefits of LifeWave patches to promote healing, enhance energy, alleviate pain, and improve sleep quality. As we delve deeper into the healing power of light, LifeWave Patch Therapy leads the way in this fascinating journey toward wellness.

Benefits of Using LifeWave Patches
LifeWave Patch Therapy is known for its many advantages, providing a gentle,

drug-free way to improve health and well-being. LifeWave patches utilize phototherapy technology to encourage the body's own healing processes, boost energy levels, ease pain, and enhance sleep—all while avoiding the use of chemicals or medications. This section will explore the many benefits of LifeWave patches, such as their potential to enhance healing, naturally increase energy levels, alleviate chronic pain, and promote better sleep quality.

Finding Wellness with Gentle Approaches

One of the most appealing aspects of LifeWave Patch Therapy is how it encourages healing in a gentle, non-invasive way. In contrast to traditional treatments that typically rely on medications, injections, or surgeries, LifeWave patches tap into the body's natural healing abilities through the use of light. These options appeal to individuals looking for natural remedies or those who may feel uncertain about pursuing more intense treatments.

LifeWave patches work by utilizing phototherapy, a method that harnesses light to encourage particular biological reactions within the body. The patches are applied to the skin at particular acupuncture points, where they engage with the body's natural infrared heat to reflect certain wavelengths of light. These light signals activate biochemical responses that encourage healing within our cells. Some LifeWave patches are created to encourage the production of stem cells, which are essential for healing and regenerating tissues.

What makes LifeWave patches unique compared to other healing methods is that they are non-transdermal. This indicates that the skin and bloodstream do not absorb anything—healing processes are triggered solely by light. This approach helps to lower the chances of experiencing side effects that people often face with medications, like allergies, irritations, or negative interactions between drugs. This approach enables people with sensitive skin or weakened immune systems to enjoy the therapy, alleviating worries about bringing foreign substances into their bodies.

LifeWave patches can also be paired with other treatments, like physical therapy or chiropractic care, to support the body's healing journey. These have proven effective in helping people recover after surgery, rehabilitate from sports injuries, and manage chronic conditions such as arthritis and tendonitis. LifeWave patches can support quicker healing and lessen recovery time, allowing people to get back to their everyday lives sooner and with less discomfort.

Naturally Increasing Your Energy Levels

One of the most valued advantages of LifeWave Patch Therapy is its capacity to enhance energy levels in a natural way. Numerous individuals face challenges with fatigue and low energy, often stemming from stress, inadequate nutrition, insufficient sleep, or ongoing health issues. Unlike traditional options that rely on caffeine, stimulants, or energy drinks, LifeWave patches provide a natural and sustainable way to boost energy, helping you feel more vibrant without the jitters or crashes.

The Energy Enhancer patch stands out as a favorite among the offerings in the LifeWave line. This product aims to boost your energy and stamina by enhancing how your body produces energy at the cellular level. The patch helps by improving circulation, boosting oxygen levels, and aiding the body in turning food into energy more effectively. By applying the Energy Enhancer patch to certain acupuncture points, the body can tap into its resources more efficiently, resulting in a significant boost in energy and stamina.

The secret to enhancing energy with LifeWave patches is rooted in the fascinating science of light and its impact on our cells. LifeWave patches work by energizing the mitochondria, the cell's powerhouses, leading to a boost in the production of adenosine triphosphate (ATP). This molecule plays a crucial role in storing and transferring energy within our cells. When ATP levels are elevated, cells can carry out their tasks more effectively, leading to a boost in energy levels across the body.

What makes LifeWave patches an attractive choice for enhancing energy is their natural approach. They avoid using artificial stimulants or chemicals, which can create issues like dependency, tolerance, or negative side effects. LifeWave patches align with the body's natural energy systems, offering a gentle and lasting boost that enhances overall vitality. These options are great for athletes aiming to boost their performance, busy professionals wanting to increase their productivity, or anyone dealing with chronic fatigue in need of sustained energy support.

Additionally, LifeWave patches work harmoniously with the body's natural circadian rhythms and sleep patterns, ensuring they are a safe choice for daytime use without the worry of affecting your sleep. Many people share that they feel more awake, concentrated, and lively during the day, without experiencing the jitters or energy dips that are usually linked to caffeine or other stimulants.

Finding Relief from Chronic Pain Without Medications

Chronic pain impacts countless individuals around the globe, resulting in a diminished quality of life and a greater dependence on pain relief medications. Sadly, traditional pain relief methods can bring about considerable drawbacks, such as the potential for addiction, developing tolerance, and experiencing side effects. LifeWave Patch Therapy provides a fresh approach to pain relief that is gentle, non-invasive, and free from addictive substances or pharmaceuticals.

The IceWave patch is crafted to provide relief from pain and has become a trusted choice for individuals dealing with chronic pain conditions like arthritis, fibromyalgia, back pain, and joint discomfort. The IceWave patch, when placed on certain areas of the body, utilizes phototherapy to help reduce inflammation, enhance circulation, and ease pain by focusing on the body's natural pain pathways. Many users find that they feel quick relief just minutes after applying the patches, making them a helpful choice for managing both sudden and ongoing pain.

One of the significant benefits of using LifeWave patches for pain relief is that they focus on the root cause of pain instead of just covering up the symptoms. Unlike traditional pain medications that simply block pain signals to the brain, LifeWave patches work with the body to reduce inflammation and encourage healing, offering a path to long-lasting relief. This natural approach reduces the reliance on medications, which can lead to unwanted side effects such as drowsiness, stomach problems, or dependency.

LifeWave patches offer the advantage of being safely integrated with other pain management approaches, including physical therapy, acupuncture, or chiropractic care. Numerous individuals share that LifeWave patches boost the effectiveness of these treatments, helping them lessen their dependence on medications or invasive procedures.

For individuals dealing with conditions such as arthritis or tendonitis, marked by inflammation and ongoing discomfort, LifeWave patches offer a gentle yet effective approach to symptom management. The patches work to ease inflammation and support tissue healing, allowing users to enjoy improved mobility and comfort without relying on medications.

Enhancing Sleep Quality

In our busy lives today, many people are experiencing sleep disturbances more often. Lots of individuals find it challenging to drift off, maintain their slumber, or reach that deep, restorative sleep. There are many sleep aids you can find, both over-the-counter and prescription, but they often bring along some unwanted side effects like feeling groggy, becoming dependent, or experiencing issues with thinking clearly. LifeWave Patch Therapy provides a gentle, non-invasive way to enhance sleep quality, allowing the body to naturally manage its sleep-wake cycle without relying on medications.

The Silent Nights patch aims to help you achieve better sleep by boosting your body's natural melatonin production, the hormone that plays a key role in regulating your sleep cycle. As evening approaches and darkness sets in, melatonin levels usually increase, gently signaling to our bodies that it's time to wind down and embrace sleep. Yet, things like stress, being around artificial light, and having inconsistent sleep routines can throw off melatonin production, resulting in insomnia or less restful sleep. Using the Silent Nights patch can gently encourage your body to produce melatonin, making it easier to drift off to sleep, stay asleep throughout the night, and experience a more refreshing rest.

The Silent Nights patch stands out because it offers a natural way to enhance sleep quality. The Silent Nights patch offers a different approach compared to traditional sleep aids. Instead of simply sedating the brain or causing drowsiness, it aligns with the body's natural circadian rhythms, encouraging a more organic and restorative sleep experience. This helps minimize the chances of feeling groggy the next day or experiencing a sleep hangover that some medications can cause.

Along with enhancing how long and well you sleep, LifeWave patches might also tackle some of the root causes of sleep problems, like pain, stress, or anxiety. Users often share that after using the patches for pain management or stress relief, they notice a significant enhancement in their ability to enjoy a restful night's sleep. This comprehensive approach to sleep health makes LifeWave patches a great choice for those looking for lasting solutions to sleep issues without depending on medications or artificial supplements.

LifeWave Patch Therapy provides a gentle, non-invasive way to enhance health and wellness using the principles of phototherapy. If you're looking for natural methods to increase your energy, ease chronic pain, or enhance your sleep quality, LifeWave patches offer a safe, drug-free option that helps activate your body's own healing processes. LifeWave patches have gained popularity among those seeking to naturally enhance their quality of life, thanks to their ability to promote healing, boost vitality, and offer lasting relief.

CHAPTER 1

Understanding Phototherapy and Its Mechanism

What is Phototherapy?

Phototherapy, also known as light therapy, is a time-honored healing practice that has transformed into a contemporary therapeutic method utilized for numerous medical and wellness applications. Phototherapy, with its rich history and modern advancements like LifeWave Patch Therapy, uses the power of light energy to encourage healing, restore balance in the body, and enhance overall well-being. This chapter explores the basics of phototherapy, tracing its roots, examining how light engages with the body to create healing effects, and highlighting the main distinctions between conventional phototherapy and LifeWave's unique method.

Understanding Phototherapy

Phototherapy is a healing approach that harnesses light energy to encourage recovery, ease discomfort, and enhance overall wellness. Phototherapy is based on a straightforward idea: light, as a form of energy, can interact with our bodies and affect different biological processes. Certain wavelengths of light can reach the skin and interact with cells, tissues, or organs, initiating a series of reactions that result in therapeutic advantages.

For thousands of years, people have used phototherapy in different ways. Ancient civilizations understood the healing power of sunlight, harnessing its warmth and light to address various health issues, from skin problems to uplifting spirits. Today, phototherapy has grown to encompass a variety of light-based treatments, including full-spectrum light therapy as well as focused laser and LED therapies. LifeWave Patch Therapy offers a distinctive, gentle method of phototherapy that harnesses the body's own infrared energy to reflect particular light wavelengths, supporting health and healing.

The Story Behind Phototherapy

Phototherapy has roots in ancient civilizations that recognized the natural healing abilities of light. The ancient Egyptians, Greeks, and Romans all engaged in some form of heliotherapy, which is the therapeutic use of sunlight. In ancient Egypt, sunlight was viewed as a sacred source of healing, with medical texts from that time detailing its use in treating a range of ailments, especially skin diseases. In Greece, the philosopher Herodotus encouraged sunbathing as a way to regain health, while the Romans created solaria, dedicated spaces for soaking up the sun.

In the more recent past, the healing power of light found its footing in the scientific community during the 19th century, thanks to Danish physician Niels Ryberg Finsen, who pioneered the first medical use of phototherapy. In the late 1800s, Finsen found that specific wavelengths of light could help treat diseases such as skin tuberculosis (lupus vulgaris). His groundbreaking contributions to ultraviolet light therapy led to him receiving the Nobel Prize in Medicine in 1903, representing a major achievement in the exploration of light therapy.

Since then, phototherapy has evolved, benefiting from improvements in laser technology, light-emitting diodes (LEDs), and full-spectrum lamps. Today, light therapy is utilized to address various conditions, such as seasonal affective disorder (SAD), psoriasis, wound healing, chronic pain, and even sleep disorders. The continuous study of how light impacts our biology has given rise to creative solutions such as LifeWave Patch Therapy, which harnesses light in a distinctive manner to encourage the body's inherent healing processes.

The Interaction of Light Energy with Our Bodies

To grasp the essence of phototherapy, it's important to focus on the idea of photobiomodulation—how light interacts with and influences biological functions. Light energy consists of photons, and when these photons come into contact with the skin, they can reach different depths based on the wavelength. Various wavelengths of light relate to distinct colors and can influence the body in different ways.

For instance, red light and near-infrared light can go through the skin to access muscles and tissues, helping to encourage cellular repair and lessen inflammation. Blue light, in contrast, penetrates less deeply and is frequently utilized for addressing skin issues like acne and psoriasis. The different colors of light each have their own unique way of interacting with our bodies, leading to various responses.

At the cellular level, light engages with mitochondria, the energy-producing organelles that play a vital role within our cells. When certain wavelengths of light hit the mitochondria, they kickstart the creation of adenosine triphosphate (ATP), the main molecule that stores and transfers energy in our cells. When ATP production goes up, it boosts how our cells work, speeds up tissue healing, and helps lower inflammation—each of these plays a vital role in the healing journey.

Besides boosting energy production, light can also affect the release of nitric oxide, a molecule that helps widen blood vessels and enhance circulation. Improved circulation allows for enhanced delivery of oxygen and nutrients to tissues, which helps support the body's natural healing abilities. Light therapy can also influence the activity of proteins involved in the inflammatory response, helping to ease pain and reduce inflammation.

Phototherapy can boost how our cells work, help blood flow, and ease inflammation, making it a valuable option for addressing various issues, including skin problems, chronic pain, and injuries. What makes LifeWave Patch Therapy truly special is its distinctive approach of utilizing light in a gentle, non-invasive, and drug-free manner.

Comparing LifeWave and Traditional Phototherapy

Although traditional phototherapy and LifeWave Patch Therapy both use light to aid healing, they approach the delivery of that light to the body in distinctly different ways.

1. Traditional Phototherapy: - This approach usually means letting your body soak up light from various sources, like the sun, ultraviolet (UV) lamps, infrared lights, or LED devices. These treatments take place in safe settings, like medical clinics or through at-home light therapy devices, where individuals are gently exposed to certain wavelengths of light for a set duration.
- Traditional phototherapy usually involves direct exposure to light, which can carry some risks, especially with UV-based treatments. Extended exposure to UV rays can raise the chances of skin damage, sunburn, and potentially skin cancer.
- Standard phototherapy treatments often focus on particular parts of the body and might necessitate protective gear, like goggles, to safeguard delicate areas from light exposure.

2. LifeWave Patch Therapy: - Unlike other options, LifeWave patches do not emit any light on their own. Instead, they depend on the body's own natural infrared heat to trigger the patch. The warmth from these patches reflects certain wavelengths of light back into the body, gently stimulating the photoreceptors and initiating natural biochemical processes that support healing.

- LifeWave patches are designed to be non-transdermal, which means that they do not allow any chemicals or substances to be absorbed into the skin. This offers a safer option compared to traditional light-based therapies, which can sometimes expose individuals to UV light or other irritants that may cause discomfort.

- LifeWave patches function by reflecting light instead of emitting it, making them easy to wear throughout the day. This allows users to enjoy the advantages of phototherapy seamlessly, without disrupting their everyday activities. The convenience and simplicity of LifeWave patches offer a great solution for those seeking ongoing support for pain relief, boosting energy, or improving sleep quality.

- LifeWave patches offer a range of applications. Every kind of patch serves a unique purpose, whether it's to ease inflammation, boost energy levels, or enhance sleep quality. By focusing on particular acupuncture points, LifeWave patches can offer either localized or broader effects, tailored to what the user requires.

3. Avoid Harmful Light: One of the main distinctions between LifeWave Patch Therapy and traditional phototherapy is the absence of direct light exposure in LifeWave's method. Traditional phototherapy, particularly UV-based treatments, needs careful attention to prevent overexposure, as it can lead to harmful effects. Unlike other options, LifeWave patches work with the body's natural heat and reflect light safely, which means there's no risk of skin damage or complications that can come from direct light exposure.

4. Gentle, Ongoing Care: - Phototherapy sessions typically come with constraints related to time and place, as they often necessitate a trip to a clinic or the use of a device for a designated duration. LifeWave patches can be worn for long durations, offering ongoing benefits without the hassle of frequent sessions or special equipment.

Phototherapy has a rich and intriguing history, starting from its ancient practice in heliotherapy to the contemporary uses of lasers, LEDs, and LifeWave Patch Therapy. Unlike traditional phototherapy, which depends on external light sources to trigger biological processes, LifeWave offers a fresh perspective by harnessing the body's natural infrared energy to activate patches that reflect therapeutic wavelengths of light. This special, gentle approach provides a safe and easy way to use light for healing, relieving pain, boosting energy, and enhancing sleep.

In the upcoming chapters, we will take a closer look at the unique advantages of LifeWave Patch Therapy, focusing on its potential to alleviate chronic pain, boost energy levels, and enhance sleep quality. By exploring the principles of phototherapy and recognizing how LifeWave stands apart from conventional methods, you can feel empowered to make thoughtful choices about incorporating this innovative technology into your health and wellness journey.

The Science Behind LifeWave Patches

LifeWave patches offer a unique approach to phototherapy, harnessing the body's natural energy to encourage healing from within. These patches utilize a patented technology that stands out in the realm of light therapy. LifeWave patches stand out from traditional methods because they don't need an external light source like a lamp or laser. They utilize the body's natural infrared energy to reflect specific light wavelengths back into the body, gently stimulating acupuncture points without the use of needles. This section will explore the fascinating science behind LifeWave patches, looking at how they function, their targeting of acupuncture points, and the way they encourage healing through light signals.

Innovative LifeWave Patch Technology

At the heart of LifeWave's innovation is its unique, patented patch technology that doesn't involve transdermal methods. Non-transdermal means that, unlike the usual patches used in medicine (like nicotine patches), LifeWave patches don't bring any chemicals or drugs into the body. Instead, they function by using a unique mix of organic materials incorporated into the patch, which are intended to absorb and reflect the body's infrared energy.

Each individual's body naturally gives off warmth as infrared light. LifeWave patches are made with a special crystal lattice structure that engages with infrared light. When the patches are placed on the skin, this lattice sends certain wavelengths of light back into the body. The light signals help to activate the body's own healing and regulatory processes. The material of the patch plays a vital role in how it works, influencing the kind of light it reflects. This makes the patches useful for various health benefits, including pain relief, boosting energy, or improving sleep quality.

Every LifeWave patch serves a unique function, such as the IceWave patch aimed at alleviating pain and the Energy Enhancer patch focused on boosting stamina. The unique impact of each patch arises from the specific wavelengths of light they reflect, designed to elicit different biological reactions.

This technology is truly remarkable because it can activate photoreceptors in the body without needing any external light source. The way the patch interacts with the body's infrared heat turns the body into a personal light therapy device. This feature enables therapy to be continuous and non-invasive throughout the day, allowing the patches to be worn

during everyday activities, offering ongoing benefits without disrupting the user's routine.
Exploring How LifeWave Patches Activate Acupuncture Points Without Needles

One of the most distinctive features of LifeWave patches is their capacity to activate acupuncture points without requiring needles. Traditional acupuncture focuses on harmonizing the flow of energy, known as Qi, through pathways in the body referred to as meridians. An imbalance in this energy flow can result in pain, illness, or dysfunction. Acupuncture seeks to bring harmony by gently placing fine needles at specific points along the body's pathways, encouraging the natural healing process within.

LifeWave patches provide comparable benefits without needing to penetrate the skin. When placed on certain acupuncture points, the patches activate these areas through the light reflected by the patch, which interacts with the photoreceptors in the skin. The body perceives this light as a natural signal, similar to how it responds to the physical sensation of a needle during acupuncture. This stimulation triggers a series of physiological responses, like releasing endorphins, boosting circulation, or easing inflammation, based on the specific area being addressed.

This gentle method offers a number of benefits compared to traditional acupuncture:

- Gentle Approach: It's understandable that some individuals feel uneasy about acupuncture due to the thought of needles. However, it's worth noting that the needles used in acupuncture are incredibly thin and typically result in very little discomfort. LifeWave patches offer a gentle, non-invasive way to activate acupuncture points without discomfort.
- User-Friendly: Acupuncture treatments involve going to a licensed practitioner, but LifeWave patches offer the flexibility to be used at home, on the go, or wherever you find it convenient. The patches are simple to use and can be comfortably worn under your clothes, providing ongoing therapy all day long.
- Ongoing Engagement: During a typical acupuncture session, the needles are gently placed and remain in position for about 20 to 40 minutes. LifeWave patches offer ongoing stimulation to acupuncture points for several hours, potentially extending the therapeutic benefits.

LifeWave brings together the benefits of phototherapy and acupuncture in a simple, user-friendly patch, providing an innovative option for those looking for natural healing and wellness support. The patches can be placed on various acupuncture points, tailored to the particular condition being addressed. Patches meant for pain relief can be applied to areas where muscle tension or inflammation occurs, while those intended to enhance energy levels are positioned on spots linked to vitality and stamina.

The Body's Natural Healing Journey with Light Signals

The body is a remarkable system that inherently has the capability to heal itself. LifeWave patches harness the body's natural ability to heal by utilizing light signals. The understanding of how our body reacts to light, referred to as photobiomodulation, is well established. When light meets the skin, it can go beyond the surface and influence the deeper tissues at a cellular level. Various wavelengths of light can impact the body in unique ways, and LifeWave patches are crafted to reflect certain wavelengths that are recognized for their ability to aid in healing.

1. Activation of Photoreceptors: The skin is home to unique receptors called photoreceptors that respond to light.

When the specific wavelengths of light reflected by LifeWave patches meet these receptors, they set off a chain of biochemical changes. This interaction leads to the activation of mitochondria, the tiny powerhouses within our cells that generate energy. When mitochondrial activity is boosted, cells are able to generate more adenosine triphosphate (ATP), the essential molecule that powers their functions. When there is more ATP, cells are better equipped to heal themselves, which results in quicker recovery and less inflammation.

2. Enhanced Circulation: Another way that LifeWave patches support the body's healing process is by encouraging better circulation. When specific acupuncture points are activated, either with needles or gentle light signals, the body reacts by boosting blood flow to that area. Improved circulation delivers more oxygen and nutrients to tissues, aiding in the healing process. Improving blood flow is crucial for easing pain and inflammation, as it helps remove waste products like lactic acid that can accumulate in muscles and lead to discomfort.

3. Reduction of Inflammation: Inflammation is a normal aspect of how our body defends itself, but when it

becomes chronic, it can result in pain and harm to our tissues. LifeWave patches assist in adjusting the body's inflammatory response by encouraging it to generate more anti-inflammatory substances, like cytokines. This effect works to ease swelling, pain, and discomfort, making the patches especially helpful for issues like arthritis, muscle strains, and other inflammatory conditions.

4. Balancing of the Nervous System: LifeWave patches may assist in harmonizing the autonomic nervous system, which plays a crucial role in regulating various involuntary functions in the body, such as heart rate, digestion, and responses to stress. The light signals from the patches can activate the vagus nerve, which plays a key role in soothing the nervous system and encouraging a sense of relaxation. One reason LifeWave patches work well is that they help improve sleep quality and reduce stress. The patches help promote relaxation and recovery by supporting the parasympathetic nervous system, making them a helpful resource for managing stress and addressing sleep issues.

5. Natural Pain Relief: Pain is something many people experience, and it's often a key reason why they turn to therapies

such as acupuncture or phototherapy. LifeWave patches provide a natural approach to alleviating pain by encouraging the body to release its own pain-relieving substances, like endorphins. These natural substances function like the body's own pain relievers, interrupting pain signals and offering comfort without the unwanted side effects that come with medications. LifeWave patches offer a compelling choice for individuals seeking to manage chronic pain while avoiding pharmaceuticals.

LifeWave patches offer a fresh perspective on health and wellness, blending the ideas of phototherapy and acupuncture to encourage the body's own healing abilities. These non-transdermal patches work by reflecting certain wavelengths of light, which activate photoreceptors in the skin. This process boosts cellular energy, enhances circulation, and helps reduce inflammation. Stimulating acupuncture points without needles offers a convenient and pain-free option compared to traditional therapies, enabling individuals to enjoy the advantages of light therapy anytime and anywhere.

This innovative technology provides a gentle, non-invasive solution for various health issues, including pain relief, boosting energy, enhancing sleep, and reducing stress. In the upcoming chapters, we will delve into how certain LifeWave patches can effectively address these common health concerns, providing a helpful guide for integrating LifeWave Patch Therapy into your everyday routine.

CHAPTER 2

Types of LifeWave Patches

An Overview of Different Patches

LifeWave provides a range of patches, each crafted to address unique health needs using gentle, light-based therapy. These patches help by reflecting the body's infrared energy back into the skin, encouraging natural processes that support healing, boost energy, relieve pain, improve sleep, and more. This chapter will take a closer look at the various types of LifeWave patches and how they can help with everyday health issues. These patches provide a gentle and safe alternative to medications and invasive procedures, making them an attractive choice for those looking for holistic health options.

A Look at Various Patches

LifeWave has created a variety of unique patches, with each one designed to fulfill a particular purpose. The patch system offers a range of options, enabling users to select a patch or mix and match patches that best fit their health aspirations. Let's take a closer look at some of the most popular LifeWave patches, highlighting their unique benefits and how they can be used.

X39 Patch: A Pathway to Healing and Renewal

The X39 patch is one of LifeWave's most innovative creations, aimed at helping the body's natural healing processes by activating stem cells. Stem cells are the body's essential building blocks, playing a crucial role in healing and renewing tissues. As we grow older, our stem cells become less active, which can result in slower healing, decreased energy, and a higher chance of developing age-related illnesses.

The X39 patch functions by reflecting certain wavelengths of light that encourage the body to produce GHK-Cu, a naturally occurring copper peptide recognized for its ability to activate dormant stem cells. When stem cells spring into action, they play a vital role in healing tissues, mending injuries, and enhancing our overall health. This patch has been shown to help with: - Wound healing: Stem cells play an essential role in tissue repair, which means the X39 patch can be helpful in speeding up recovery from injuries, surgeries, and wounds.

- Pain relief: Many individuals using the X39 patch share their experiences of feeling less chronic pain, which seems to stem from its potential to aid in cellular repair and lessen inflammation.

- Boosted energy and vitality: The X39 patch may help the body regenerate more effectively, potentially leading to increased stamina and overall energy levels, which can help fight the fatigue that often comes with aging.

The X39 patch is often called a anti-aging patch due to its ability to stimulate the body's natural regenerative processes. Many people are drawn to it for its potential to boost longevity, speed up recovery, and help them feel youthful as they grow older.

Energy Enhancer Patch: Elevating Your Physical Vitality

The Energy Enhancer patch aims to naturally uplift your physical energy, stamina, and endurance. This patch is perfect for athletes, fitness lovers, or anyone wanting to boost their energy levels during the day without depending on stimulants like caffeine or sugar.

This patch helps by activating certain acupuncture points linked to energy production in the body. When the reflected light from the patch activates these points, it boosts the body's metabolism, resulting in a greater production of ATP (adenosine triphosphate), which serves as the energy currency for our cells. This leads to:
- Enhanced athletic performance: Numerous individuals share experiences of boosted stamina and endurance during their workouts, leading to this patch being favored by runners, cyclists, and various endurance enthusiasts.
- Quicker recovery: The Energy Enhancer patch may help boost cellular energy production, potentially leading to shorter recovery times after intense workouts or physical exertion.
- Steady energy all day long: Unlike stimulants that give you a quick jolt followed by a slump, the Energy Enhancer patch provides reliable energy without the downsides of caffeine or other stimulants.

The Energy Enhancer patch offers a significant advantage by helping the body tap into its own natural energy production processes. This offers a better option compared to energy drinks or supplements that frequently have harmful ingredients or lead to feelings of jitteriness and anxiety.

IceWave Patch: A Natural Approach to Pain Relief

The IceWave patch is crafted to help with pain relief. It provides a gentle, drug-free, and non-invasive option for addressing both sudden and ongoing pain issues. The IceWave patch works by gently activating acupuncture points that help ease pain and reduce inflammation in the body.

One of the standout aspects of IceWave is its dual-patch system. The system features two patches—a white patch and a tan patch—that are positioned on either side of the area experiencing pain. This enables a focused energy flow, forming a circuit of relief that directly addresses the area of pain more efficiently.

Here are some of the important advantages of IceWave:
- Alleviation of chronic pain: For those dealing with arthritis, fibromyalgia, or other persistent conditions, IceWave offers enduring relief without the unwanted side effects often associated with pain medications.

- Relief from acute injuries: IceWave offers a way to ease the pain associated with sprains, muscle strains, or other injuries that often occur during sports activities.
- Completely safe: IceWave provides a safe and natural way to manage pain, standing apart from traditional pain medications that often lead to gastrointestinal problems, dependency, or other unwanted side effects.

The IceWave patch has gained a lot of attention from individuals looking for comfort from various types of pain, including back pain, joint discomfort, and muscle soreness. This provides a gentle alternative to over-the-counter painkillers or prescription medications, offering a safe and effective way for individuals to manage pain in a more natural manner.

Silent Nights Patch: Enhancing Sleep Quality

The Silent Nights patch aims to enhance sleep quality by helping the body maintain its natural sleep rhythms. In our busy lives today, many individuals face challenges with sleep, whether it's insomnia, low sleep quality, or trouble drifting off at night.

The Silent Nights patch operates by reflecting light wavelengths that engage acupuncture points associated with the regulation of the pineal gland, which plays a key role in producing melatonin— the hormone that governs our sleep-wake cycle. The Silent Nights patch helps the body naturally produce melatonin, promoting:
- Quicker to dreamland: A lot of people notice that they drift off to sleep faster when they use the Silent Nights patch.
- Better sleep experience: The patch supports users in staying asleep longer and enjoying deeper, more restorative rest, which is essential for overall health and well-being.
- Regulation of circadian rhythms: Silent Nights can be especially helpful for individuals facing challenges like jet lag, shift work, or other interruptions to their natural sleep-wake patterns.

The Silent Nights patch provides a natural way to support the body's sleep processes, serving as a drug-free option compared to sleeping pills that may leave users feeling sluggish or create a reliance. Silent Nights encourages a peaceful and restorative sleep experience, free from any unwanted side effects.

Extra Patches for Detoxification, Youthfulness, and Stress Relief

Alongside the X39, Energy Enhancer, IceWave, and Silent Nights patches, LifeWave provides a variety of other patches designed to target specific health issues. Here are some examples:

- Glutathione Patch: Created to aid detoxification by boosting the body's natural production of glutathione, a strong antioxidant that assists the liver in removing toxins. This patch is perfect for anyone wanting to boost their immune system, enhance skin health, and guard against oxidative stress.

- Carnosine Patch: Designed to enhance well-being, the Carnosine patch helps support cellular health, tissue repair, and cognitive function. It is frequently utilized to support muscle recovery, safeguard against cellular damage, and boost cognitive clarity.

- Aeon Patch: The Aeon patch is recognized for its capacity to ease stress and encourage relaxation. It supports the body's stress response by minimizing inflammation and fostering a well-balanced autonomic nervous system. This patch is perfect for anyone wanting to handle stress in a natural way, enhance mental clarity, and nurture emotional health.

LifeWave provides a wide selection of patches designed to support different areas of health and wellness. LifeWave patches, including the innovative X39 stem cell activation patch and the Silent Nights sleep patch, offer a gentle and effective approach to enhance healing, increase energy, alleviate pain, and promote better sleep without invasive procedures. Every patch is thoughtfully crafted to tap into the body's natural energy, providing a gentle and drug-free option compared to traditional treatments. If you're aiming to cleanse your body, minimize the effects of aging, or cope with stress, LifeWave offers a patch designed to support your health aspirations.

CHAPTER 3

How to Use LifeWave Patches

General Guidelines for Patch Application

LifeWave patches provide an easy and effective way to boost wellness by tapping into the body's innate healing abilities. To truly benefit from these patches, it's important to grasp the right application techniques and usage guidelines. This chapter will delve into the fundamental principles of using LifeWave patches. It will discuss the best locations for application, methods to enhance their effectiveness, and provide guidance on patch rotation and cycling.

Helpful Tips for Applying Patches

Using LifeWave patches the right way is essential for getting the best outcomes. The patches function by reflecting the body's infrared energy, gently stimulating specific acupuncture points or areas of the skin, which can lead to a range of health benefits. Although the process is simple, adhering to some essential guidelines can greatly enhance your experience.

Applying LifeWave Patches: A Guide

One of the key benefits of LifeWave patches is how they can be used in various ways. They can be used on particular acupuncture points or placed directly on the area that needs attention. Every type of patch serves a unique purpose, and the guidelines for where to place them can differ a bit based on what each patch is meant to do. Here are some helpful tips for your application:

1. Find the right acupuncture points: Each LifeWave patch includes guidance on the optimal placement for achieving the best outcomes. These places are often linked to traditional acupuncture points that are believed to affect energy flow, promote healing, and lead to specific health benefits. The Energy Enhancer patch is usually applied to the Kidney 1 and Pericardium 6 points, which are linked to enhancing energy and vitality.

2. Use on clean, dry skin: Make sure the spot where you're applying the patch is clean and dry, without any lotions, oils, or sweat. This allows the patch to stick more effectively and makes sure that the

body's infrared energy is reflected properly. Cleaning the skin with a damp cloth or an alcohol swab before applying can really help it stick better.

3. Placement over the area of concern: For pain relief patches like IceWave, it's usually helpful to position the patch right over or close to where the pain is coming from. If you're dealing with knee pain, placing the IceWave patch right on or near your knee could help you find some focused relief.

4. Consider using adhesive if necessary: LifeWave patches are typically made to adhere effectively to the skin, but some individuals might find them challenging to keep in place in humid conditions or during intense physical activities. In these situations, applying medical tape or an extra adhesive patch can effectively keep the patch securely in position.

5. Make sure to drink enough water: To help the patches perform at their best, it's essential to keep yourself well-hydrated. Staying hydrated boosts the body's conductivity and can make the patches work even better. Try to drink at least 8 glasses of water each day while using the patches.

Suggestions for Achieving the Best Outcomes

While the LifeWave patches are quite user-friendly, there are a few strategies you can adopt to enhance your experience and make the most of them. To make the most of the patches, it's essential to consider a few key factors.

1. Stick to the suggested time: LifeWave patches are meant to be worn for up to 12 hours each time you apply them. Once 12 hours have passed, it's a good idea to take off the patch so your body can have a chance to rest and reset. Using the patch for longer than suggested might lessen its effectiveness, since the skin's capacity to reflect infrared energy decreases as time goes on.

2. Apply patches regularly: To achieve the best outcomes, it's essential to use the patches on a consistent basis over time. It might take a few days or even weeks for you to start noticing improvements in your healing and overall health. Numerous LifeWave users share their experiences of slowly noticing improvements in their symptoms with consistent use. For instance, those using the Silent Nights patch for sleep might find that it takes a few nights of use

before they start to see meaningful changes in their sleep patterns.

3. Think about where to place the patches: LifeWave offers suggestions on acupuncture points, but keep in mind that everyone's body might react a bit differently to different placements. If you're not seeing the results you hoped for from one placement, it might be worth exploring a different acupuncture point or area of the body. Some users have discovered that applying the Energy Enhancer patch to the lower back yields better results compared to placing it on the ankles.

4. Combine patches for enhanced benefits: LifeWave patches can work together to tackle various health issues simultaneously. For example, you might consider using the X39 patch to support regeneration and healing, while pairing it with the Energy Enhancer patch to increase your stamina and vitality. By combining patches, you can focus on particular areas while also promoting general well-being.

5. Listen to your body: Be mindful of how your body reacts to the patches, especially when you first begin using them. Some individuals see quick benefits, while others might observe

changes that unfold more slowly over time. If you feel any discomfort or irritation where the patch is applied, consider relocating it to another spot or shortening the time you wear it.

6. Combine with healthy lifestyle choices: LifeWave patches can provide notable health benefits, and their impact can be improved when paired with a balanced diet, consistent exercise, and good sleep routines. Taking care of your body through a balanced lifestyle can enhance the effectiveness of the patches and promote your overall well-being.

Getting to Grips with Patch Rotation and Cycle

LifeWave patches are created to function gradually, and grasping the idea of patch rotation and cycling is essential for enhancing their effectiveness over the long haul. Regular rotation helps the body keep enjoying the benefits of the patches without getting used to their effects.

1. Change up where you place the patches: For patches such as the Energy Enhancer or IceWave, which are typically positioned on certain acupuncture points, it's a good idea to switch the placement site from time to time. Repeatedly using

the same site might lessen the patch's effectiveness or lead to irritation. Switching between various acupuncture points helps create a more harmonious energy flow and enhances stimulation.

2. Different patch types: Some LifeWave users switch between various patch types based on what they need at the moment. If you're mainly using the X39 patch to activate stem cells but sometimes deal with pain, you could try switching between the X39 patch on certain days and the IceWave patch on others. Using alternating patches can offer well-rounded support for various health objectives, all while avoiding excessive stimulation of any single system.

3. Adhere to suggested patch cycles: For specific patches, it can be helpful to implement them in cycles. Some LifeWave users might choose to wear the Glutathione patch daily for detoxification for a period of 5 days, taking a break for 2 days afterward. This cycle allows the body to take a breather and rejuvenate, helping the patch to function better over time.

4. Apply at certain times of day: Some patches might be more effective when used at particular times. For instance,

the Silent Nights patch is meant to help with sleep and is best applied before you go to bed to achieve optimal results. On the other hand, the Energy Enhancer patch is ideally used in the morning or early afternoon to help boost your stamina and vitality as you go about your day.

5. Take breaks when necessary: Although the patches are made to be safe for daily use, some individuals might benefit from taking occasional breaks, particularly after using the patches for several weeks consecutively. This allows the body to take a breather and helps avoid any potential dulling of the patches' effects.

Understanding how to use LifeWave patches correctly and following their guidelines is essential for getting the most out of them. Using the patches for pain relief, boosting energy, or enhancing sleep? By following these best practices, you can get the most out of them and see steady improvements in your health. By following proper placement techniques, staying hydrated, rotating patches, and using them in cycles, you can help your body's natural healing processes and enhance your overall wellness with the benefits of phototherapy.

LifeWave Patches and Acupressure Points

LifeWave patches aim to encourage the body's natural healing processes by utilizing light energy that interacts with particular acupressure or acupuncture points. These patches offer a gentle approach, eliminating the need for needles or chemicals, and serve as a non-invasive alternative to traditional acupuncture. To get the most out of LifeWave patches, it's important to know the key acupressure points and how to place the patches correctly. This section delves into how acupressure points play a part in LifeWave patch therapy, offering clear, step-by-step guidance for proper placement to address a range of health issues, including pain relief, energy enhancement, better sleep, and detoxification.

Important Acupressure Points for Various Health Benefits

Acupressure, much like acupuncture, revolves around the idea of energy pathways, or meridians, that flow through our bodies. By gently stimulating certain points along these meridians, we can positively affect the flow of energy, or Qi, which helps in healing, alleviating pain, and enhancing our overall sense of well-being. LifeWave patches, when applied to these important acupressure points, support the body's innate healing capabilities. Here are some of the acupressure points that people often use for different health benefits.

1. Finding Comfort

The IceWave patch is often utilized for alleviating pain. IceWave is crafted to help ease inflammation and provide relief by placing it on targeted acupressure points or right over the painful area.

- Li4 (Large Intestine 4): Often referred to as the Union Valley, this point can be found in the webbing between your thumb and index finger. Gently working on this area can bring comfort from headaches, toothaches, and overall body discomfort.

- St36 (Stomach 36): This point, referred to as Leg Three Miles, can be found four finger widths beneath the kneecap and roughly one finger width toward the outside of the leg. St36 is known for its strong ability to relieve pain, particularly in the legs, knees, and back.

- Sp6 (Spleen 6): This point is found roughly three finger widths above the inner ankle bone. Known as the Three

Yin Intersection, it is commonly used to help ease menstrual discomfort, digestive problems, and lower back pain.

Patch Placement: - IceWave Patches: Place one patch on Li4 and the other on Sp6 to create a strong synergy for pain relief. Another option is to apply one patch right on the area where you're feeling pain and place the second patch nearby for targeted relief.

2. Elevating Your Energy

The Energy Enhancer patch is designed to boost energy and stamina by activating acupressure points that help enhance the body's natural energy flow. These patches can be applied to specific areas that stimulate energy pathways, enhancing circulation and overall vitality.

- Ki1 (Kidney 1): Found on the sole of the foot, in the little dip just below the ball, Kidney 1, often called Bubbling Spring, serves as a grounding point that helps enhance energy flow throughout the body. This aspect supports kidney health and enhances overall well-being.

- PC6 (Pericardium 6): Often referred to as Inner Gate, this point can be found roughly two finger widths above the wrist on the inner forearm. By focusing on this point, you may find a boost in energy, a decrease in nausea, and a clearer mind.

- GV20 (Governing Vessel 20): Found at the crown of the head, this point is known as the Hundred Meeting Point. It helps boost alertness and energy by activating the body's governing meridian.

Patch Placement: - Energy Enhancer Patches: Put the patches on Ki1 for an impressive energy boost. Another option is to position them on PC6 to boost mental clarity and stamina. To enhance your experience, consider trying out the patches on GV20 to help with overall energy balance.

3. Enhancing Sleep Quality

The Silent Nights patch aims to support better sleep by soothing the nervous system and encouraging a sense of relaxation. This patch is applied to acupressure points that help relieve stress and improve sleep quality.

- Yintang (Third Eye Point): Found between the eyebrows, this point is known to help ease stress, soothe the mind, and encourage improved sleep. It's often called the Hall of Impression.

- Anmian (Peaceful Sleep Point): Located just behind the ear, in the small dip between the base of the skull and the mastoid bone, Anmian is an important point in Traditional Chinese Medicine that helps with insomnia and enhances sleep quality.

- HT7 (Heart 7): Referred to as Spirit Gate, this spot can be found at the wrist crease on the inner forearm, aligned with the pinky finger. HT7 is often utilized to soothe the mind and encourage a peaceful night's sleep.

Patch Placement: - Silent Nights Patch: Place the patch on the Yintang point to promote a soothing experience that helps you drift off into a restful sleep. Another option is to place the patch behind the ear on the Anmian point to help improve your sleep patterns. If you're dealing with anxiety-related sleep problems, trying the patch on HT7 might help soothe your mind and improve your sleep quality.

4. Cleansing and Easing Tension

The Glutathione and Y-Age Aeon patches are well-liked for their roles in detoxification and providing stress relief, respectively. These patches support the body in fighting oxidative stress and removing toxins, all while encouraging a sense of relaxation and overall well-being.

- LIV3 (Liver 3): This point, often referred to as Great Rushing, is situated on the top of the foot, nestled between the first and second toes. This point in acupuncture is known for its strong ability to help detoxify the body, particularly by clearing toxins from the liver and providing a sense of stress relief.

- LI11 (Large Intestine 11): Found at the outer end of the elbow crease, this point, often referred to as Pool at the Crook, is recognized for its role in clearing heat from the body, supporting detoxification, and alleviating inflammation.

- Gallbladder 34 (GB34): Located on the side of the leg, just below the knee, GB34, known as Yang Mound Spring, plays an important role in helping to clear the body's meridians and support detoxification, particularly for the liver and gallbladder.

Patch Placement: - Glutathione Patch: Apply the patch on LIV3 to help with detoxification and enhance liver function. Another option is to place the patch on LI11, which can assist in clearing heat from the body and improving detoxification.

- Y-Age Aeon Patch: For stress relief, place the patch on GB34 to help clear energetic blockages and encourage a soothing effect. Using the Glutathione and Y-Age Aeon patches together can offer enhanced detoxification and help alleviate stress.

Guidelines for Applying Your Patch

Getting the patch placement just right is essential for maximizing the benefits of LifeWave patches. Take a moment to go through these steps to make sure you're applying the patches the right way:

1. Prepare Your Skin: Make sure your skin is clean, dry, and free from any lotions, oils, or sweat before putting on the patch. This helps the patch stick properly and allows the skin's infrared energy to be effectively reflected by it.

2. Find the Acupressure Point: Refer to diagrams or guides to pinpoint the specific acupressure point that aligns with your health objective. If you're looking to relieve pain, consider locating points such as LI4 or Sp6 that can help with that purpose.

3. Remove the backing and place the patch: Take the LifeWave patch out of its packaging, carefully peel off the adhesive backing, and place the patch right onto the selected acupressure point. Make sure it is securely fastened to the skin.

4. Check in on Comfort and Effectiveness: After applying the patch, take note of how your body feels and reacts. Some users notice changes right away, while others might see improvements over time. If you're experiencing any discomfort or irritation, try relocating the patch to a different spot.

5. Take Off After 12 Hours: LifeWave patches are meant to be used for a maximum of 12 hours. Once the time is up, take off the patch and throw it away. Please avoid reusing patches, as they lose their effectiveness after being used once.

6. Hydrate: It's essential to drink enough water while using LifeWave patches. Staying hydrated supports your body's energy and enhances the effectiveness of the patches.

The effectiveness of LifeWave patch therapy greatly relies on the proper placement of patches on important acupressure points. When you're looking to ease pain, increase your energy, enhance your sleep, or support detoxification, knowing the right spots and methods for applying these patches is essential. By following the steps outlined above, you can enhance the healing potential of LifeWave patches and tap into your body's natural energy for improved health and well-being.

CHAPTER 4

Healing with LifeWave Patches

Using LifeWave Patches for Healing

LifeWave patches provide a distinctive and gentle approach to encourage healing, speed up tissue repair, and assist the body's natural detoxification efforts. These patches utilize phototherapy, a method that employs light-based energy transfer to target specific points on the skin, helping to activate the body's natural healing processes. LifeWave patches offer a natural way to enhance health without relying on drugs or invasive procedures, making them an attractive option for anyone looking for holistic healing solutions.

This chapter will delve into the ways LifeWave patches can help speed up tissue repair, lessen inflammation, aid in healing minor wounds and injuries, and assist the body in its detoxification efforts. Every one of these functions plays a part in enhancing our physical health and overall well-being.

Utilizing LifeWave Patches for Recovery

LifeWave patches are crafted to align with the body's natural functions, supporting the healing of damaged tissues and helping to ease inflammation. Healing is a complex journey that includes the renewal of cells, strengthening the immune system, and clearing out toxins. LifeWave patches offer therapeutic benefits across these areas, creating a holistic approach to healing.

1. Speeding Up Tissue Healing and Easing Inflammation

Inflammation is a normal part of how our bodies heal, but when it becomes chronic, it can slow down tissue repair and cause ongoing discomfort. LifeWave patches may assist in lessening inflammation and promoting the healing of tissues by encouraging the body's innate healing processes.

- Stem Cell Activation (X39 Patch): The X39 patch is crafted to stimulate stem cells, which play a vital role in the body's natural healing process for damaged tissues. Stem cells play a vital role in creating new cells that can take the place of those that have been harmed or lost due to injury. The X39 patch works by activating these cells, helping to speed up tissue regeneration and enhance the healing process.

Clinical studies indicate that X39 patches can help lessen inflammation, a common factor that can slow down the healing process. The patch, when placed on an injury or inflamed area, can gently stimulate certain points, helping to improve circulation and boost the flow of oxygen and nutrients to the affected tissue. This process helps to speed up healing while also easing pain and reducing swelling.

- Minimizing Oxidative Stress (Y-Age Aeon Patch): Another important aspect of tissue repair is minimizing oxidative stress, as it can hinder healing by harming cells and tissues. The Y-Age Aeon patch is designed to reduce oxidative stress in the body, helping to lessen cellular damage and inflammation. This patch helps your body by encouraging the release of natural antioxidants. These antioxidants play a crucial role in shielding you from free radicals, which are harmful molecules that can worsen inflammation and slow down the healing process.

How to Use: - To support tissue repair, you can place the X39 patch on the GV14 point (found on the upper spine) or the CV6 point (just below the navel). Both of these areas are recognized for their healing benefits. To help with localized inflammation, try placing the X39 patch close to the injury site. You might also think about adding the Y-Age Aeon patch to help reduce inflammation and oxidative stress even more.

2. Caring for Minor Wounds, Injuries, and Cuts

LifeWave patches are helpful for addressing minor injuries like cuts, bruises, and sprains. The patches support quicker tissue repair and lessen inflammation, making the healing process more comfortable and efficient for wounds.

- IceWave for Comfort: The IceWave patch can be really helpful for easing pain from injuries such as sprains or muscle strains. In contrast to traditional pain relief options that rely on medications, IceWave employs light therapy to gently alleviate pain and inflammation in a natural way. This method stimulates specific acupuncture points, helping to block pain signals and encouraging the release of endorphins, which are the body's natural pain relievers.

For issues like a muscle strain, joint pain, or a small wound, the IceWave patch can be applied right on or close to the painful spot, offering relief without the unwanted side effects of medications.

- Aiding in the Recovery of Cuts and Bruises: Using LifeWave patches on cuts or bruises may help to enhance the healing process. The X39 and IceWave patches work together to help ease inflammation and support the growth of new tissue, which can assist in healing wounds and restoring bruised or damaged skin.

- Enhancing Circulation for Quicker Recovery: When circulation is poor, it can slow down the healing process of wounds and injuries by limiting the delivery of oxygen and nutrients to the area in need. LifeWave patches enhance circulation by encouraging the flow of energy throughout the body's meridians, aiding in the delivery of vital nutrients to injured tissues. This improved blood flow helps you recover more quickly.

How to Use: - For cuts and minor wounds, place the X39 patch close to the injury to help stimulate stem cell regeneration. To help with pain from injuries, position the IceWave patch on opposite sides of the painful area. This can create a flow of energy that eases your discomfort. Consider pairing the patches for a combined benefit—X39 to support healing and IceWave for alleviating pain.

3. Helping the Body Cleanse Itself

Detoxification plays a vital role in healing, as getting rid of toxins and waste from the body is crucial for our cells to function well and repair themselves. LifeWave patches are important for helping the body detox naturally by boosting the functions of the liver, kidneys, and other organs involved in detoxification.

- Glutathione Patch for Detox: The Glutathione patch stands out as a favored choice among LifeWave patches for detoxification. Glutathione is a remarkable antioxidant that helps to neutralize toxins, lessen oxidative stress, and bolster the immune system. The patch supports the body in producing more glutathione, which in turn helps to speed up the elimination of harmful substances from within.

When toxins accumulate in the body, they can disrupt how our cells function and hinder the healing process. The patch works to boost glutathione levels, aiding in the detoxification of the liver, kidneys, and lymphatic system, which play a crucial role in filtering and removing toxins from the body. This helps in healing and also protects tissues and cells from future harm due to the buildup of toxins.

- Y-Age Carnosine Patch for Cellular Detox: The Y-Age Carnosine patch offers a way to help support detoxification right at the cellular level. Carnosine is a natural molecule that plays a vital role in safeguarding our cells from oxidative damage while boosting their self-repair capabilities. This patch enhances the health of individual cells, helping the body detoxify more effectively and improving the overall healing process.

How to Use: - For detoxification support, place the Glutathione patch on the LIV3 point (located on the foot between the big and second toes) to boost liver function. To enhance cellular detox, apply the Y-Age Carnosine patch on ST36 (located just below the kneecap on the outer side of the leg), recognized for its detoxification advantages.

Using LifeWave patches for healing offers a gentle and natural way to tap into the body's own energy systems, helping to speed up recovery, lessen inflammation, and aid in detoxification. By gently activating acupuncture points with light therapy, LifeWave patches can help speed up tissue healing, ease discomfort, and support the body's natural detoxification processes, all without relying on medications or invasive procedures.

If you're facing an injury, trying to ease chronic inflammation, or wanting to cleanse your body, LifeWave patches offer a safe, effective, and drug-free way to support healing and enhance your overall well-being. When used correctly, these patches can be a valuable addition to your wellness journey, supporting you in achieving improved results and quicker recovery from various health challenges.

CHAPTER 5

Boosting Energy Levels Naturally

Energy Enhancement with LifeWave Patches

Energy forms the core of our well-being and liveliness. Lacking enough energy can lead to a drop in both physical and mental performance, making it hard for the body to operate at its best. Many people struggle with chronic fatigue, feeling drained, or lacking energy for a variety of reasons, such as their lifestyle choices, stress, or health issues that may be lurking beneath the surface. Unlike traditional methods for boosting energy, like caffeine or energy drinks, which can give you a quick lift but often lead to a crash, LifeWave patches provide a more natural and sustainable approach. They work by harnessing the body's own energy production systems to enhance your energy levels.

This chapter explores how LifeWave patches, especially the Energy Enhancer patch, can naturally elevate energy levels by promoting ATP production, improving physical stamina, and helping to combat chronic fatigue. We will delve into the science behind these patches, looking at how they affect cellular energy and the advantages they offer to everyone, from regular individuals to athletes.

Boost Your Energy with LifeWave Patches

LifeWave patches operate through phototherapy, using particular wavelengths of light to encourage the body's natural energy production processes. The Energy Enhancer patch is crafted to boost the body's natural energy production at a cellular level, all without relying on stimulants or medications.

These patches work by stimulating acupressure points that are linked to energy production, helping to enhance physical stamina, endurance, and overall vitality. LifeWave's approach to energy enhancement focuses on nurturing the body's inherent capacity to generate and maintain energy all day long, rather than just offering temporary solutions.

1. The Role of Patches in Boosting ATP Production and Cellular Energy

At the heart of how our bodies produce energy is a molecule known as

Adenosine Triphosphate (ATP), which serves as the energy currency for our cells' activities. Every cell in our body depends on ATP to perform its essential functions, whether it's helping our muscles move or supporting our thinking processes. When the body can produce and use ATP more effectively, energy levels rise.

- LifeWave and ATP Production: LifeWave patches, especially the Energy Enhancer patch, activate important acupressure points that boost the body's ATP production. In contrast to stimulants that give a temporary energy lift, LifeWave patches enhance the body's natural energy processes by boosting mitochondrial function, which is crucial for producing ATP in our cells.

Clinical studies have indicated that individuals using the Energy Enhancer patch often notice marked improvements in their energy levels and metabolic efficiency. Applying the patches to certain meridian points helps to enhance the body's energy flow. This leads to improved oxygen use, more effective fat burning, and a boost in ATP production. This journey results in increased energy and improved overall stamina.

- Improving Mitochondrial Performance: The mitochondria, commonly known as the powerhouses of our cells, are the places where ATP is created. When mitochondria are working well, they can generate more energy, and LifeWave patches are important for maintaining mitochondrial health. These patches utilize light therapy to activate energy-related acupoints, enhancing mitochondrial efficiency and enabling cells to generate more ATP with reduced effort. You'll notice a boost in your energy levels that lasts all day long.

How to Use: - For optimal ATP production, you can place the Energy Enhancer patches on specific points like SP6 (found on the inner leg, a few inches above the ankle) or LI4 (located on the hand between the thumb and index finger), both of which are recognized for their ability to enhance energy and vitality. You can use the patches every day or whenever you feel the need to help boost your cellular energy production.

2. Boosting Physical Stamina and Endurance for Athletes

No matter if you're a professional athlete or just someone who loves to play sports for fun, having physical stamina and endurance is crucial for how well you perform. Feeling fatigued, experiencing muscle weakness, and struggling with endurance can really affect how well athletes perform and how quickly they recover. LifeWave patches, particularly the Energy Enhancer, provide a natural approach to enhancing physical performance by optimizing energy metabolism, oxygen use, and endurance.

- Enhancing Oxygen Use: Oxygen plays a vital role in how well athletes perform. The way our bodies use oxygen plays a crucial role in how effectively our muscles work when we engage in physical activities. LifeWave patches support the body by enhancing oxygen uptake and boosting circulation, leading to improved stamina and endurance. Athletes are able to sustain their performance for extended durations without feeling tired as soon as they might otherwise.

Studies have indicated that the Energy Enhancer patch can help the body metabolize fat and carbohydrates more effectively, offering a better fuel source for prolonged physical activity. When the body becomes more efficient at metabolism, athletes are able to access their energy reserves better, which results in improved performance and quicker recovery.

- Enhancing Muscle Function and Recovery: LifeWave patches boost energy levels and aid in improving muscle function during exercise. By targeting specific acupressure points that promote energy flow, the patches assist muscles in contracting more efficiently, potentially boosting strength, endurance, and recovery.

For athletes, taking time to recover is just as crucial as their performance on the field. After a tough workout, our muscles require time to heal and grow stronger. LifeWave patches, like the Energy Enhancer, can help with muscle recovery by improving circulation and minimizing lactic acid buildup, which often leads to soreness and fatigue.

How to Use: - For boosting stamina and endurance, athletes can place the Energy Enhancer patches on points such as ST36 (just below the knee) or K1 (on the sole of the foot), which are recognized for their potential to enhance energy and endurance. To achieve the best results, it's a good idea to apply the patches before engaging in physical activity. This helps your body get ready for optimal performance.

3. Battling Chronic Fatigue and Low Energy

Feeling constantly tired and lacking energy is something many people experience. It can often stem from stress, not getting enough sleep, not eating well, or even hidden health issues. LifeWave patches provide a natural way to tackle fatigue and boost energy levels by encouraging the body's own energy production pathways.

- Support for Chronic Fatigue Syndrome (CFS): Chronic Fatigue Syndrome (CFS) is marked by a deep and lasting fatigue that doesn't seem to get better, even with rest. Individuals dealing with CFS frequently experience diminished mitochondrial function and challenges in energy production. LifeWave patches provide a natural approach to help manage and ease the symptoms of chronic fatigue by enhancing ATP production and improving energy flow.

Using Energy Enhancer patches on certain acupressure points can help people feel more energized, think more clearly, and lessen their fatigue. These patches help bring harmony to the body's energy systems, promoting a more consistent energy flow throughout the day.
- Supporting Mental Energy: Feeling mentally drained can be just as challenging as feeling physically tired.

LifeWave patches offer a boost to your physical energy while also enhancing your mental clarity and focus. The Energy Enhancer patch, when placed on energy-boosting acupressure points, supports brain function, alleviates brain fog, and improves cognitive performance. This serves as a helpful resource for individuals facing challenges with mental fatigue or focus issues.

- Navigating Everyday Challenges: Stress plays a significant role in causing fatigue and low energy levels. LifeWave patches assist the body in managing stress by nurturing the parasympathetic nervous system, the part that promotes relaxation and recovery. Using patches to stimulate acupressure points can help soothe the nervous system, allowing people to enhance their ability to handle stress and keep their energy levels up throughout the day.

How to Use: - If you're dealing with chronic fatigue or low energy, try applying the Energy Enhancer patch to points like PC6 (located on the inner forearm) or GV20 (found on the top of the head). These spots can help boost your vitality and improve mental clarity. For individuals experiencing chronic fatigue, these patches can be incorporated into a daily routine as a long-term approach to enhance energy levels and overall well-being.

LifeWave patches provide a natural and effective way to enhance energy levels, increase stamina, and fight off fatigue. These patches tap into the body's natural energy production systems, offering a sustainable and enduring source of energy without the unwanted side effects associated with stimulants or medications. If you're aiming to boost your athletic performance, tackle chronic fatigue, or just elevate your everyday energy, LifeWave patches offer a valuable resource for enhancing both physical and mental well-being.

The Energy Enhancer patch helps you produce more ATP, use oxygen more effectively, and enhance your overall endurance, making it a great addition to your health and wellness routine. When you learn to use these patches in the right way, you can connect with your body's natural energy, leading to increased energy levels, enhanced performance, and a better overall quality of life.

Improving Focus and Mental Clarity

In our busy lives today, staying focused and keeping a clear mind is crucial like never before. No matter if you're a student, a professional, or a caregiver, being able to focus and think clearly is crucial for your productivity, creativity, and overall well-being. LifeWave patches provide a natural and effective method to boost cognitive function and enhance mental clarity through the use of phototherapy.

This chapter will delve into how LifeWave patches can aid in boosting cognitive function, sharpening focus, and keeping you energized all day long. Let's explore the science behind these patches, how they affect mental performance, and practical ways to enhance your cognitive abilities.

LifeWave Patches and How They Affect Our Thinking

Cognitive function encompasses a range of mental processes, such as attention, memory, reasoning, and problem-solving. Various elements can affect how well we think and perform mentally, such as stress, tiredness, what we eat, and distractions in our surroundings.

LifeWave patches, especially those aimed at boosting energy and enhancing mental clarity, can offer valuable support for cognitive function through their distinctive mechanisms.

1. Boosting Brain Function with LifeWave Patches

LifeWave patches use a blend of light therapy and acupressure to activate particular points on the body. This stimulation can help boost brain function and enhance how we think and learn.

- Enhancing Neurotransmitter Function: Neurotransmitters are the brain's chemical messengers, essential for regulating our mood, enhancing focus, and ensuring cognitive clarity. LifeWave patches may support the production of important neurotransmitters like dopamine and serotonin, which are linked to better mood and heightened focus. By activating specific areas on the body that influence these neurotransmitters, individuals might find improved focus, less mental exhaustion, and a greater feeling of wellness.

- Enhancing Circulation to the Brain: Good blood circulation is vital for our brains to work at their best. LifeWave patches support circulation, enhancing the flow of oxygen and nutrients to the brain. Better blood flow can help you think more clearly, stay alert, and perform better mentally. Many users share that they feel more awake and focused after using the patches, which helps them approach their tasks with improved efficiency.

- Encouraging Calmness and Easing Tension: Elevated stress can hinder our thinking abilities and contribute to mental exhaustion. LifeWave patches support the body in finding its relaxation response, fostering a feeling of calm and easing anxiety. When people manage their stress, they can enhance their focus and gain better mental clarity. The Silent Nights patch can assist in regulating sleep patterns and improving the quality of rest, which in turn can enhance cognitive performance during waking hours.

How to Use: For boosting cognitive function and mental clarity, simply place the Energy Enhancer patch on acupressure points like GV20 (found at the top of your head) or PC6 (located on the inner forearm). These points are recognized for their ability to enhance brain function and boost mental alertness.

2. Keeping Your Energy Up All Day Long
The levels of energy we have can significantly influence how well we think and how clear our minds feel. When energy levels dip, it can be tough to focus, think clearly, and maintain productivity. LifeWave patches offer a natural way to enhance your energy and keep your focus sharp all day long.

- Consistent Energy Flow: Unlike typical energy enhancers such as caffeine, which often result in sudden spikes and drops in energy, LifeWave patches provide a more stable and continuous energy experience. These patches support the body by boosting ATP production and enhancing mitochondrial function, allowing for a more efficient use of energy reserves. This leads to a consistent flow of energy, helping people stay focused and involved in what they're doing.

- Tackling Afternoon Slumps: A lot of us feel a dip in energy during the afternoon, which can make it tough to stay focused and productive. LifeWave patches offer a way to naturally enhance your energy levels and tackle this issue. Using the Energy Enhancer patch in the mid-afternoon can help people recharge their energy and boost mental clarity, enabling them to tackle the remainder of the day with renewed vigor.

- Caring for Your Brain's Nutritional Needs: Good nutrition is essential for how our minds work. LifeWave patches can support a healthy diet by improving the body's capacity to absorb and make use of nutrients vital for brain health. Nutrients such as omega-3 fatty acids, B vitamins, and antioxidants play a vital role in supporting brain function, and LifeWave patches may enhance the efficiency of these important processes.

How to Use: To keep your energy levels steady all day long, simply place the Energy Enhancer patch on at the start of your day or when you feel that afternoon dip. Applying the patches to important acupressure points can enhance energy levels and boost cognitive function. It's important for users to pay attention to a balanced diet full of nutrients to really get the most out of the patches.

Enhancing focus and mental clarity is essential for reaching success in different areas of life. LifeWave patches provide a natural and effective approach to boosting cognitive function, supporting brain health, and keeping your energy levels up all day long. These patches work by harnessing the power of light and gentle pressure to activate important points in the body. This process helps boost neurotransmitter activity, improve blood flow, and encourage a sense of calm.

If you're aiming to boost your mental clarity, keep your energy levels up throughout a hectic day, or alleviate stress-induced tiredness, LifeWave patches can offer the assistance you're seeking. By using these patches regularly and applying them correctly, you can tap into your cognitive abilities, allowing you to concentrate more effectively, think with greater clarity, and approach challenges with fresh energy and mental sharpness.

CHAPTER 6

Pain Relief through LifeWave Patch Therapy

Effective Pain Management

Pain is something we all go through, touching the lives of countless people around the globe. Managing pain effectively is essential for preserving our quality of life, whether it's from injury, chronic conditions, or the everyday strains and stresses we all face. Conventional approaches to managing pain frequently depend on medications that may result in undesirable side effects and potential dependence. LifeWave patches, especially the IceWave patch, provide a gentle, non-invasive option for pain relief, helping people take charge of their health and well-being.

This chapter delves into the use of LifeWave patches for managing pain effectively, with a particular emphasis on the IceWave patch for addressing both acute and chronic pain. We'll also talk about ways to ease muscle soreness, joint pain, and headaches, and look into how to blend LifeWave therapy with other natural methods for pain relief.

Compassionate Pain Relief with LifeWave Patches

Managing pain includes a variety of methods, from medications to physical therapies and changes in daily habits. LifeWave patches offer a distinctive way to find relief from pain by using phototherapy and acupressure, enabling users to enjoy considerable comfort without the dangers linked to conventional pain medications.

1. Utilizing IceWave for Both Acute and Chronic Pain

The IceWave patch is thoughtfully crafted to deliver quick and effective relief from pain. This approach combines light therapy and acupressure to encourage the body's natural healing abilities, providing relief from both acute and chronic pain.

- Mechanism of Action: IceWave patches function by reflecting certain wavelengths of light that reach the skin and activate acupressure points. This stimulation can help your body release endorphins, which are its natural pain-relieving chemicals, and enhance blood flow to the area that needs it most. Consequently, many people find that their pain and inflammation decrease, which makes IceWave a helpful option for anyone dealing with different kinds of pain.

- Immediate Pain Relief: Sudden pain, often caused by injury or trauma, can be overwhelming. IceWave patches can be placed right on the area where you're feeling pain to help you feel better right away. For instance, someone with a sprained ankle can apply the patch to the hurt area to help ease swelling and discomfort. Numerous users share that they experience significant benefits just minutes after using the patches, enabling them to get back to their usual activities sooner.

- Chronic Pain Management: Living with chronic pain, which is pain that persists for more than three months, can be quite difficult to navigate. Conditions like arthritis, fibromyalgia, and lower back pain frequently need continuous care approaches. LifeWave patches can easily fit into everyday life, offering ongoing comfort and support. Using IceWave patches on specific acupressure points linked to pain can help individuals feel a noticeable decrease in discomfort as time goes on.

How to Use: For quick relief from pain, place IceWave patches directly on the area that hurts or around it, based on what kind of pain you're experiencing. For managing chronic pain, individuals can alternate the patches on and off the painful area or place them on acupressure points recognized for their pain-relieving properties, like LI4 (found between the thumb and index finger) or SP6 (a few inches above the ankle).

2. Easing Muscle Discomfort, Joint Aches, and Headaches

LifeWave patches offer a flexible solution for easing different kinds of discomfort, such as muscle soreness, joint pain, and headaches.

- Muscle Soreness: Following a tough workout or physical activity, you might experience muscle soreness, which happens because of tiny tears in your muscle fibers. IceWave patches can be placed on sore muscles to help ease inflammation and support quicker recovery. These patches can help ease discomfort and boost flexibility by improving blood flow and minimizing lactic acid buildup.

A study involving athletes found that those who used IceWave patches experienced notable decreases in muscle soreness and faster recovery times than those who didn't use the patches. The patches offered quick relief while also helping the body heal naturally, allowing athletes to push their limits and bounce back more quickly.

- Joint Pain: Conditions such as osteoarthritis and rheumatoid arthritis can cause ongoing joint pain that disrupts everyday life. IceWave patches can be really helpful for easing joint pain, offering targeted support to sore joints. When users apply the patches to the affected joints, they frequently notice less pain and a boost in their ability to move around.

Using IceWave patches regularly may assist in managing chronic joint pain, which can lessen the reliance on over-the-counter pain medications and their possible side effects. People can also pair the patches with gentle exercises or stretches to boost joint mobility and comfort even more.

- Headaches: Headaches and migraines can really affect how we go about our day-to-day activities. LifeWave patches may offer relief by placing IceWave patches on certain acupressure points linked to headache alleviation, like GB20 (found at the base of the skull) or Yintang (situated between the eyebrows). Numerous individuals share that applying IceWave patches to these areas can provide relief from headache symptoms in just a few minutes.

How to Use: To ease muscle soreness, place the IceWave patch right on the affected area after your workout. To help with joint pain, apply the patches around the sore joint, making sure to cover it well. To relieve headaches, apply IceWave patches to specific acupressure points and let them sit for about 20-30 minutes to achieve the best results.

3. Merging LifeWave with Other Natural Approaches to Alleviate Pain

LifeWave patches are not only effective on their own, but they can also be seamlessly incorporated into a broader pain management strategy that embraces other natural therapies. Using LifeWave patches alongside other supportive methods can improve pain relief and foster a sense of overall well-being.

- Physical Therapy and Exercise: Adding physical therapy or gentle exercise to a pain management routine can greatly enhance results. LifeWave patches offer quick pain relief, while physical therapy works to build muscle strength, enhance flexibility, and reduce the risk of future injuries. Applying IceWave patches before and after physical therapy sessions can ease discomfort and aid in the recovery process.

- Massage Therapy: Massage offers a wonderful opportunity to ease muscle tension and encourage a sense of relaxation. Using LifeWave patches alongside massage therapy can lead to improved pain relief. Using IceWave patches on sore spots before a massage can enhance the therapist's ability to work effectively. These patches help alleviate pain and inflammation, making it possible for deeper tissue work to be done without causing discomfort.

- Herbal Remedies: Some herbal remedies, like turmeric and ginger, offer anti-inflammatory benefits that can work well alongside LifeWave patches. Adding these herbs to your meals can help with managing pain more effectively. For instance, savoring a turmeric latte or ginger tea while applying IceWave patches can support your body's natural healing abilities.

- Practices for Mindfulness and Relaxation: Stress and tension can make pain feel even worse. Using mindfulness practices like meditation, yoga, or deep-breathing exercises can be a gentle way to manage pain by encouraging relaxation. Incorporating LifeWave patches into these practices can truly enrich the experience, fostering deeper relaxation and providing more effective pain relief.

How to Use: For the best pain relief experience, think about pairing LifeWave patches with additional approaches that suit your individual needs. If you're using IceWave patches for joint pain, consider incorporating some light stretching or yoga to help improve your flexibility and range of motion.

LifeWave patch therapy provides a meaningful and effective way for people to find relief from pain, helping them to handle both acute and chronic discomfort in a natural manner. The IceWave patch offers focused relief for different kinds of pain, such as muscle soreness, joint discomfort, and headaches, all while avoiding the side effects that often come with conventional medications.

By learning to use LifeWave patches effectively and pairing them with other natural pain relief techniques, people can develop a well-rounded approach to managing pain that enhances their overall health and wellness. LifeWave patches give individuals the ability to manage their pain and enhance their overall well-being, enabling them to participate fully in everyday activities without the constraints of discomfort.

CHAPTER 7

Better Sleep with LifeWave Patch Therapy

The Silent Nights Patch for Restful Sleep

Sleep is essential for our health and well-being, but many people find it challenging to get the restful and restorative sleep they need. Things like stress, anxiety, lifestyle choices, and health issues can really throw off our sleep, causing insomnia and other sleep problems. LifeWave patches, especially the Silent Nights patch, provide a distinctive and effective way to enhance sleep quality and duration, assisting people in regaining their peaceful nights.

In this chapter, we will delve into the significance of sleep, the fascinating science of circadian rhythms and sleep cycles, and how LifeWave patches can improve the quality of your rest. We'll also talk about how the Silent Nights patch can help with sleep issues, like insomnia and interrupted sleep.

The Silent Nights Patch for a Peaceful Sleep

The Silent Nights patch is thoughtfully crafted to encourage relaxation and foster healthy sleep habits. This patch offers a gentle, non-invasive way for people looking to enhance their sleep quality, using the principles of phototherapy and acupressure.

1. Getting to Know Your Body's Natural Rhythms and Sleep Patterns

Understanding the body's circadian rhythms and sleep cycles is key to appreciating the impact of LifeWave patches on sleep.

- Circadian Rhythms: These are the natural internal processes that help manage our sleep-wake cycle and other bodily functions throughout a 24-hour day. These rhythms are shaped by outside factors like light and temperature, and they are essential in guiding our feelings of alertness and fatigue. When our natural body clocks get thrown off, it can result in sleep problems and various health concerns.

- Sleep Stages: Sleep consists of various stages, such as light sleep, deep sleep, and REM (rapid eye movement) sleep. Every stage comes with its own distinct traits and roles:

- Light Sleep (Stage 1 and 2): This early phase of sleep plays a crucial role in helping us move from being awake to entering deeper sleep. At this stage, the body starts to unwind, the heart rate eases, and muscle activity lessens.
- Deep Sleep (Stage 3): Often referred to as slow-wave sleep, deep sleep plays a vital role in helping our bodies restore themselves, support tissue growth, and boost immune function. This phase of sleep is truly essential, as it's when our bodies take the time to heal and recharge, helping us feel our best.
- REM Sleep: This stage plays a crucial role in our cognitive abilities, helping us consolidate memories, learn new things, and manage our emotions effectively. It features quick eye movements and heightened brain activity.

When our natural sleep patterns are thrown off, it can really affect how well we sleep. This often leads to feeling tired, cranky, and not thinking as clearly as we'd like.

2. The Impact of Phototherapy on Sleep Quality and Duration

LifeWave patches harness the power of light through phototherapy, a method designed to enhance healing and support overall well-being. The Silent Nights patch uses this technology to improve how well and how long you sleep.

- Encouraging Calmness: The Silent Nights patch aims to encourage a sense of calm by gently stimulating acupressure points linked to relaxation and peace. Applying the patch to certain areas on the body helps activate the relaxation response, easing stress and anxiety that can disrupt sleep. This relaxation response aids in reducing cortisol levels, which is known as the stress hormone, and supports the body in moving into a more restful state.

- Managing Melatonin Levels: Melatonin is a hormone made by the pineal gland that plays a key role in managing our sleep-wake cycles. The Silent Nights patch could support your body's natural melatonin production, making it easier to drift off to sleep and stick to a regular sleep routine. LifeWave patches can assist people in promoting their body's natural hormone production, leading to healthier sleep patterns.

- Enhancing Sleep Depth and Quality: Many individuals using the Silent Nights patch frequently share their experiences of better sleep depth and quality. Using phototherapy alongside acupressure could assist individuals in reaching deeper, more restorative sleep by encouraging smoother transitions into the deep sleep stages. Getting better sleep can help you wake up feeling more refreshed and full of energy.

How to Use: For better sleep quality, simply place the Silent Nights patch on acupressure points like Yintang (found between the eyebrows) or PC6 (located on the inner forearm) around 30-60 minutes before you go to bed. This pre-sleep app helps your body unwind, making it simpler to drift off to sleep.

3. Patches for Sleep Issues: Trouble Falling Asleep and Interrupted Rest

Sleep disorders like insomnia and interrupted sleep can really affect how we experience life. LifeWave patches offer a natural option for those facing these challenges.

- Insomnia: Insomnia involves struggles with falling asleep, staying asleep, or waking up too soon. People dealing with insomnia often find themselves feeling more anxious and stressed, which can make it tough to unwind and drift off to sleep. The Silent Nights patch offers a gentle way to help manage insomnia, encouraging relaxation and supporting a healthier sleep-wake cycle. People have shared that they've noticed better sleep, finding it easier to drift off and stay asleep all night long.

- Disrupted Sleep Patterns: Things like shift work, travel, and changes in daily routines can throw off our natural sleep cycles, resulting in sleep that feels broken and unrefreshing. The Silent Nights patch is designed to help bring harmony back to your sleep cycle by encouraging relaxation and aiding in melatonin production. People have discovered that regularly using the patch can help them create more consistent sleep routines, leading to better overall sleep quality.

- Complementary Approaches: LifeWave patches can work well on their own, but they can also be paired with other natural practices that promote better sleep. Keeping a regular sleep routine, engaging in relaxation techniques, and setting up a comfortable sleep space can really boost the benefits of the patches. People might find it helpful to include herbal remedies that are recognized for their soothing properties, like chamomile or valerian root.

How to Use: If you're struggling with insomnia or have trouble sleeping, consider applying the Silent Nights patch each night, preferably 30-60 minutes before you head to bed. Creating a soothing pre-sleep routine can really help improve your sleep. Try dimming the lights, cutting back on screen time, and doing some relaxation exercises to wind down before bed.

Getting restful and restorative sleep is crucial for our health and well-being, but many people face challenges with sleep disorders and irregular sleep patterns. The Silent Nights patch provides a gentle and effective way to enhance your sleep quality and duration, utilizing the soothing principles of phototherapy and acupressure.

When we recognize how vital circadian rhythms and sleep cycles are, we can truly value the way LifeWave patches enhance our sleep experience. Using the Silent Nights patch regularly can support relaxation, boost melatonin production, and lead to better sleep quality. Integrating LifeWave therapy into a comprehensive approach to sleep management allows people to regain restful nights, which can significantly improve their physical and mental well-being.

Techniques to Maximize Sleep Quality

Getting restorative sleep is essential for your physical health, mental well-being, and overall quality of life. LifeWave patches, especially the Silent Nights patch, can be a great aid in enhancing sleep quality. When paired with good sleep hygiene practices and helpful lifestyle tips, their effectiveness can be further improved. In this section, we will look at helpful techniques to enhance sleep quality, allowing everyone to experience deeper, more restorative rest.

1. Enhancing Sleep with LifeWave Patches and Healthy Habits

Sleep hygiene involves a collection of practices and habits that help ensure you get consistent, uninterrupted, and restful sleep. Combining these practices with LifeWave patches can greatly enhance sleep quality.

a. Creating a Regular Sleep Routine

Staying consistent is essential for keeping our body's internal clock in check. Going to bed and waking up at the same time each day, even on weekends, supports your body's natural rhythms, making it simpler to drift off to sleep and rise feeling rejuvenated.

- Technique: Apply the Silent Nights patch each night around 30-60 minutes before you plan to go to sleep. This pre-sleep app can help you relax and gently remind your body that it's time to settle down for the night. With time, this steady routine will help your body naturally get ready for sleep.

b. Establishing a Soothing Bedtime Ritual

Taking part in soothing activities before bedtime can gently remind your body that it's time to unwind and get ready for a good night's sleep. Establishing a calming routine can help ease stress and anxiety, allowing for a smoother transition into sleep.

- Technique: Add the Silent Nights patch to your nightly routine for a more restful sleep. Use it on acupressure points like Yintang (between the eyebrows) or PC6 (on the inner forearm) while you take part in calming activities. Think about incorporating deep breathing exercises, gentle stretching, or meditation to promote relaxation.

c. Enhancing Your Sleep Space

Making your space comfortable for sleep is key to getting the best rest possible. Elements like light, noise, temperature, and comfort are crucial for encouraging a good night's sleep.

- Technique: Make your bedroom a cozy retreat by keeping it dark, quiet, and cool. Consider using blackout curtains, earplugs, or white noise machines if you find it helpful. As you get ready to settle in for the night, apply the Silent Nights patch to enhance your sleeping environment. Its soothing effects will work hand in hand with your efforts to create a tranquil space.

d. Reducing Screen Time Before Sleep

The blue light from screens can disrupt melatonin production, which can make it more challenging to drift off to sleep. Cutting back on screen time before bed can really make a difference in how well you sleep.

- Technique: Try to step away from electronic devices for at least an hour before you go to sleep. Try to immerse yourself in soothing activities like getting lost in a good book or embracing mindfulness practices. Take advantage of the Silent Nights patch during this period to encourage relaxation, helping your mind to let go of the day's events.

e. Engaging in Relaxation Techniques

Adding relaxation techniques to your nightly routine can really improve the quality of your sleep. Engaging in activities like mindfulness meditation, deep breathing, and progressive muscle relaxation can really soothe both your mind and body.

- Technique: Blend your relaxation methods with the Silent Nights patch for the best results. While you engage in mindfulness or deep breathing, pay attention to the comforting feelings from the patch, letting it deepen your tranquility and get you ready for a restful night.

2. More Lifestyle Tips for Enhanced Rest

Along with sleep hygiene practices, various lifestyle factors can affect how well we sleep. Using these tips can really boost the healing benefits of LifeWave patches.

a. Thoughtful Approaches to Eating and Drinking

Your daily choices about what you eat and drink can really affect how well you sleep at night. Some foods and drinks can help you unwind, while others might interfere with your sleep.

- Technique: Try to steer clear of heavy meals, caffeine, and alcohol as bedtime approaches. If you're feeling a bit hungry, consider having a light snack like a banana, yogurt, or a small handful of nuts. These options can help you unwind and get your body ready for a good night's sleep.

- Hydration: It's important to keep yourself hydrated, but try to watch how much you drink in the evening so you can get a good night's sleep without too many bathroom breaks. Think about enjoying herbal teas that are known to promote calmness, like chamomile or valerian root tea, before bedtime to help you unwind.

b. Consistent Movement

Getting regular exercise can help you drift off to sleep more quickly and experience a more restful night. Engaging in exercise can help alleviate stress and anxiety, two frequent obstacles to achieving a good night's sleep.

- Technique: Try to get in at least 30 minutes of moderate exercise on most days, ideally earlier in the day. After exercising in the evening, give your body a little time to cool down before heading to bed. Combine your physical activity with the Silent Nights patch after your workout to enhance recovery and promote relaxation.

c. Navigating Stress and Anxiety

Living with chronic stress and anxiety can really take a toll on how well we sleep. Adding stress management techniques to your daily routine can make it easier to overcome obstacles to getting a good night's sleep.

- Technique: Make it a habit to engage in stress-reducing activities like yoga, tai chi, or journaling. Try the Silent Nights patch during these activities to help you unwind and feel more at ease. Also, think about trying mindfulness meditation or guided imagery before you go to bed to help soothe your mind and get ready for a good night's sleep.

d. Embracing Natural Light Throughout the Day

Getting natural light is really important for keeping our body clocks in sync.

Getting some sunlight during the day helps your body know when it's time to be awake and when it's time to rest.

- Technique: Try to spend at least 20-30 minutes outside each day, particularly in the morning light. This practice supports healthy sleep patterns and can enhance the quality of your rest. In the evening, try to reduce your exposure to artificial light to help your body recognize its natural signals for sleep.

e. Assessing Sleep Position and Comfort

Your sleeping position can really influence how well you rest at night. Making sure your mattress and pillows offer the right support can really boost your comfort and help you enjoy a good night's sleep.

- Technique: Take a moment to assess your sleep environment and make sure it promotes a peaceful night's rest. Consider getting a mattress and pillows that provide the support you need based on how you sleep. As you get cozy in bed, apply the Silent Nights patch and let its soothing effects guide you gently into a restful sleep.

Improving sleep quality requires a thoughtful approach that blends good sleep habits with changes in daily routines. Integrating LifeWave patches, especially the Silent Nights patch, into a well-rounded sleep plan can help people relax more, enjoy deeper sleep, and minimize disruptions.

Having a regular sleep schedule, winding down with a calming bedtime routine, making your sleep space cozy, and using helpful relaxation methods are all important parts of taking care of your sleep health. By embracing mindful eating habits, engaging in regular physical activity, managing stress, and getting plenty of natural light, people can actively work towards enjoying deeper, more restorative sleep.

When people focus on getting enough sleep and make use of LifeWave patches, they can improve their health, feel better overall, and enjoy life more, waking up each morning feeling refreshed and energized.

CHAPTER 8

Supporting General Wellness with LifeWave Patches

Anti-Aging and Skin Health
As we grow older, our bodies experience different changes that can influence our overall health and well-being. People often look for ways to stay youthful, enhance their skin health, and boost their overall well-being. LifeWave patches provide a unique way to boost your vitality and rejuvenation using gentle, non-invasive phototherapy. This chapter will delve into how LifeWave patches can aid in anti-aging and enhance skin health, emphasizing skin rejuvenation, collagen production, and cell renewal.

1. LifeWave Patches and Skin Renewal

Taking care of your skin is an important part of feeling good and being healthy. The skin acts as a shield for our bodies, helps keep our temperature in check, and plays an important role in how we present ourselves to the world. As we grow older, our skin can lose some of its elasticity, become drier, and may be more susceptible to blemishes and wrinkles. LifeWave patches can be important for supporting skin rejuvenation by encouraging healthy cellular function and enhancing overall skin vitality.

a. The Importance of Light for Healthy Skin

LifeWave patches use the principles of phototherapy, applying light to encourage natural biological processes. Light therapy has demonstrated a range of positive effects on the skin, such as:

- Improved Blood Flow: Phototherapy boosts circulation to the skin, providing vital nutrients and oxygen while helping to eliminate waste products. Better circulation can lead to a more vibrant complexion and increased skin health.

- Encouraging Skin Healing: Light energy has the ability to reach deep into the skin, helping to activate the body's natural repair processes and support the renewal of damaged skin cells. This process may help soften the look of fine lines, wrinkles, and other signs of aging.

- Lowering Inflammation: Ongoing inflammation can play a role in different skin issues, such as acne and rosacea.

LifeWave patches may assist in reducing inflammation, leading to a calmer, clearer complexion.

b. Targeted Solutions for Skin Wellness

Some LifeWave patches are especially beneficial for promoting skin health and rejuvenation:

- X39 Patch: The X39 patch aims to activate stem cells, helping to support tissue regeneration and repair. Using the X39 patch on acupressure points might help people enjoy better skin elasticity and see fewer fine lines and wrinkles.

- IceWave Patch: The IceWave patch may help ease pain and reduce inflammation, potentially offering relief for individuals dealing with skin issues tied to inflammation, like psoriasis or eczema.

- Energy Enhancer Patch: The Energy Enhancer patch can boost energy levels, helping users feel more vibrant and motivated to stay active, which in turn supports healthy skin.

2. Encouraging Collagen Growth and Cell Regeneration

Collagen is an essential protein that gives our skin its structure and flexibility. As we grow older, our bodies produce less collagen, which can result in sagging skin, wrinkles, and a decrease in firmness. LifeWave patches may help boost collagen production and promote cell renewal, which are important for maintaining youthful skin.

a. Grasping the Role of Collagen and Why It Matters

Collagen is the most plentiful protein in our bodies, making up a large part of our skin, tendons, ligaments, and various other connective tissues. It serves important functions in keeping the skin healthy:

- Support and Elasticity: Collagen plays a vital role in giving the skin its shape and strength, contributing to its smoothness and ability to bounce back.

- Moisture Retention: Collagen plays a vital role in keeping the skin hydrated, leading to a fresh and plump look.

- Wound Healing: Collagen plays a vital role in healing wounds, aiding in the repair of damaged skin and tissue.

As we age and our collagen production decreases, many people look for ways to help boost its creation. LifeWave patches may contribute to this journey.

b. The Role of LifeWave Patches in Boosting Collagen Production

LifeWave patches have the ability to encourage the body's own healing mechanisms, supporting collagen production and improving skin health:

- Improving Cellular Interaction: LifeWave patches use light energy to activate acupressure points, promoting better communication among cells. Better communication can lead to more effective collagen production and repair processes.

- Enhancing Nutrient Uptake: The patches can help boost blood flow, which in turn may improve the delivery of vital nutrients to your skin. Vitamins and minerals like vitamin C, zinc, and amino acids play an essential role in collagen synthesis, while improved circulation helps these nutrients reach the skin more efficiently.

- Promoting a Healthy Lifestyle: The boost in energy and vitality from LifeWave patches can inspire people to make healthier choices that enhance skin health, like staying active and eating a balanced diet.

c. Cell Renewal and Skin Regeneration

LifeWave patches not only promote collagen production but also support cell renewal, contributing to a more youthful appearance of the skin.

- Boosting Skin Cell Renewal: LifeWave patches help encourage the skin's natural process of shedding old cells and generating fresh, new ones. This process may lead to a more radiant complexion and help diminish the look of fine lines and dark spots.

- Supporting Wound Healing: LifeWave patches utilize phototherapy to boost the body's inherent ability to heal wounds, helping to speed up recovery from cuts, abrasions, and various skin injuries. This skill in healing skin can lead to a healthier, more youthful look.

3. Holistic Methods to Nurture Skin Wellness

LifeWave patches provide notable advantages for skin rejuvenation and collagen production. When paired with additional supportive methods, they can further improve results and contribute to overall wellness.

a. Nourishing Choices

A balanced diet filled with vitamins, minerals, and antioxidants can really help keep your skin healthy. Think about adding foods that support collagen production and help your skin renew itself:
- Vitamin C: Present in citrus fruits, strawberries, and leafy greens, vitamin C plays a crucial role in the production of collagen.

- Healthy Fats: Omega-3 fatty acids present in fish, walnuts, and flaxseeds play a vital role in keeping skin hydrated and supple.

- Antioxidants: Enjoying foods like berries, nuts, and dark chocolate, which are packed with antioxidants, can be a delightful way to support your skin and fight oxidative stress.

b. Staying Hydrated

Keeping yourself well-hydrated is essential for ensuring your skin stays elastic and retains moisture. Make it a goal to enjoy plenty of water during your day, and think about incorporating hydrating foods such as cucumbers and watermelon into your meals.

c. Protecting Your Skin from the Sun

Too much sun can speed up the aging of your skin and harm collagen. Take care of your skin by using sunscreen every day, dressing in protective clothing, and finding shade when the sun is at its strongest.

d. Consistent Skincare Practice

Having a consistent skincare routine that involves cleansing, exfoliating, and moisturizing can really support the health of your skin. Seek out products featuring ingredients recognized for their ability to boost collagen production, like retinol and hyaluronic acid.

e. Managing Stress

Living with chronic stress can negatively impact your skin, contributing to issues such as acne and signs of aging appearing earlier than they should. Using stress management techniques like mindfulness, yoga, or meditation can support a clearer complexion and enhance overall well-being.

LifeWave patches provide a valuable resource for enhancing overall wellness, especially when it comes to anti-aging and skin health. Using the principles of phototherapy, LifeWave patches can help rejuvenate the skin, boost collagen production, and support cell renewal, leading to a more youthful and vibrant look.

By combining LifeWave patches with a well-rounded approach that embraces balanced nutrition, proper hydration, sun protection, and effective stress management, people can enhance their skin health and overall wellness. Adopting these practices can bring about a refreshed look, boost self-esteem, and enrich overall well-being, helping people to age with grace and keep their energy alive.

Balancing Hormones and Reducing Stress

Maintaining hormonal balance is crucial for our overall health and well-being, affecting aspects like our mood, energy levels, metabolism, and reproductive health. When our hormones are out of balance, it can cause a range of health challenges, such as anxiety, weight gain, fatigue, and issues related to reproduction. In our busy lives today, stress plays a big role in making hormonal imbalances worse. LifeWave patches provide a distinctive way to tackle these challenges by promoting hormonal balance and alleviating stress. This section delves into the ways LifeWave patches can affect hormonal balance while supporting emotional well-being and alleviating stress.

1. The Impact of LifeWave Patches on Hormonal Balance

LifeWave patches use the principles of phototherapy to gently stimulate specific acupressure points in the body, helping to modulate hormonal levels and support overall hormonal balance. This is how they function:

a. Grasping Hormonal Imbalance

Hormones act as chemical messengers that help manage various functions in our bodies. When hormone levels are out of balance, it can result in a range of health issues, such as:

- Menstrual Irregularities: Changes in hormones can lead to irregular periods, discomfort from cramps, and various other menstrual symptoms.

- Mood Disorders: Changes in hormones such as estrogen, progesterone, and testosterone can result in mood swings, anxiety, and feelings of depression.

- Weight Gain: Hormonal imbalances can influence how our bodies process food and regulate hunger, which may result in gaining weight and finding it challenging to shed those extra pounds.

- Fatigue: When hormone levels drop, especially thyroid hormones, it can lead to persistent tiredness and a lack of energy.

LifeWave patches may assist in restoring hormonal balance by interacting with the body's natural signaling processes and encouraging homeostasis.

b. How It Works

LifeWave patches function by using particular light frequencies to activate acupuncture points, helping to boost the body's innate healing abilities. The ways in which LifeWave patches can affect hormonal balance include:

- Improving Cellular Interaction: The light from LifeWave patches can boost the interaction between cells, encouraging a balanced release of hormones. This effect can help the endocrine system, which plays a crucial role in producing and regulating hormones.

- Stimulating Acupuncture Points: By focusing on particular acupressure points linked to hormonal balance, LifeWave patches can encourage the release of hormones such as insulin, cortisol, and sex hormones (estrogen, progesterone, and testosterone). Patches applied to the PC6 (pericardium 6) point can assist in balancing stress hormones, fostering a feeling of tranquility.

- Boosting Blood Flow: Enhanced circulation from using LifeWave patches helps ensure that hormones are effectively distributed throughout the body. This improved circulation can help the adrenal glands, thyroid, and reproductive organs work better, all of which are essential for keeping our hormones in balance.

c. Targeted Patches for Hormonal Harmony

Some LifeWave patches can be especially helpful for supporting hormonal balance:

- X39 Patch: This innovative patch is crafted to stimulate stem cells, potentially enhancing hormonal balance and boosting overall energy and well-being.

- Energy Enhancer Patch: This patch boosts energy levels, helping you lead a more active lifestyle, which is essential for maintaining hormonal health.

- Silent Nights Patch: Improved sleep quality can support the balance of hormones influenced by stress and anxiety. The Silent Nights patch may help enhance sleep patterns, which can, in turn, support hormonal balance.

2. Nurturing Emotional Well-Being and Easing Stress

Living with chronic stress can really affect your hormonal balance and how you feel overall. High cortisol levels can lead to a range of health issues, such as increased appetite, weight gain, anxiety, and trouble sleeping. LifeWave patches provide a gentle way to help manage stress and promote emotional well-being.

a. Understanding the Link Between Stress and Hormones

When we experience stress, our bodies kick into gear with a natural fight or flight response, leading to the release of hormones like cortisol and adrenaline.

123

Although these hormones play a crucial role in helping us navigate immediate stress, enduring stress can result in lasting hormone imbalances. Some typical impacts of stress on hormonal health are:

- Higher Cortisol Levels: Ongoing stress can raise cortisol levels, which may lead to feelings of anxiety, weight gain, and a weakened immune system.

- Disrupted Reproductive Hormones: Stress can throw off the balance of sex hormones, which may result in irregular periods, a drop in libido, and challenges with fertility.

- Impaired Thyroid Function: Ongoing stress can take a toll on how the thyroid works, resulting in feelings of tiredness, weight changes, and shifts in mood.

LifeWave patches may assist in easing these effects by encouraging relaxation, lowering stress levels, and helping to restore hormonal balance.

b. How LifeWave Patches Help Relieve Stress

LifeWave patches may help ease stress in a few different ways:

- Encouraging Relaxation: Using LifeWave patches can help foster a sense of relaxation and tranquility, which can be beneficial in managing the body's stress response. For instance, applying the Silent Nights patch to acupressure points can help create a sense of relaxation, which can make it simpler to handle stress.

- Boosting Mood: LifeWave patches have the potential to uplift mood and support emotional wellness. Patches can promote the release of feel-good hormones such as serotonin and dopamine, which may help ease feelings of anxiety and depression.

- Enhancing Sleep Quality: Quality sleep plays a vital role in our emotional health and helps us manage stress effectively. Utilizing LifeWave patches for better sleep can help reduce stress, boost your mood, and promote a healthier hormonal balance.

c. Targeted Solutions for Stress Relief

Some LifeWave patches can be especially helpful for enhancing emotional well-being and easing stress.

- Silent Nights Patch: This patch is crafted to enhance your sleep experience and encourage a sense of calm. Getting better sleep can really help reduce cortisol levels, making it a vital part of managing stress.

- Energy Enhancer Patch: Boosting energy levels can help fight off fatigue and lift your spirits. This patch encourages physical activity, acting as a natural way to help relieve stress.

- X39 Patch: This patch supports the activation of stem cells and boosts overall vitality, which can lead to improved emotional well-being and greater resilience to stress.

3. Lifestyle Strategies to Enhance LifeWave Patches

LifeWave patches offer valuable support for hormonal balance and stress relief, and adding complementary lifestyle strategies can boost their effectiveness:

a. Consistent Physical Activity

Engaging in physical activity is a powerful method for managing stress and achieving hormonal balance. When you exercise, your body releases endorphins, which are natural hormones that make you feel good, and this can also help lower cortisol levels.

- Technique: Try to get in at least 30 minutes of moderate exercise on most days of the week. Engaging in activities such as yoga, walking, and swimming can really help in managing stress effectively.

b. Nourishing Choices

A balanced diet filled with whole foods can nurture hormonal health and enhance emotional well-being. Foods rich in nutrients can help keep blood sugar levels steady, lower inflammation, and supply important vitamins and minerals.

- Technique: Aim to include a variety of lean proteins, healthy fats, whole grains, fruits, and vegetables in your meals. Eating foods that are high in omega-3 fatty acids, like fatty fish and flaxseeds, can be beneficial for reducing inflammation and promoting brain health.

c. Mindfulness and Relaxation Techniques

Bringing in mindfulness practices like meditation, deep breathing, and progressive muscle relaxation can really help ease stress and foster emotional balance.

- Technique: Set aside a few minutes each day to engage in mindfulness or meditation practice. Think about incorporating the Silent Nights patch during these sessions to promote relaxation and ease stress.

d. Restful Sleep

Getting quality sleep is essential for keeping our hormones in check and handling stress effectively. Establishing a regular sleep routine, along with incorporating LifeWave patches, can greatly improve the quality of your sleep.

- Technique: Establish a soothing bedtime routine, and apply the Silent Nights patch 30-60 minutes prior to sleep to encourage relaxation.

e. Community Connections

Building and nurturing meaningful relationships can greatly influence our emotional well-being. Connecting with caring friends and family can ease stress and lift your spirits.

- Technique: Set aside moments for social activities that uplift your spirit and help you unwind, whether it's joining a club, attending gatherings, or just enjoying the company of those you care about.

LifeWave patches provide a gentle, non-invasive way to help balance hormones and alleviate stress. These patches use the principles of phototherapy to help balance hormones and enhance emotional well-being. By improving how cells communicate, activating acupressure points, and encouraging relaxation, LifeWave patches can significantly contribute to achieving hormonal balance.

When paired with supportive lifestyle choices—like staying active, eating well, practicing mindfulness, and getting good sleep—LifeWave patches can boost their benefits and contribute to overall well-being. Focusing on hormonal health and managing stress can lead to enhanced vitality, emotional balance, and a better overall quality of life.

CHAPTER 9

Frequently Asked Questions and Troubleshooting

Common Questions About LifeWave Patches

When people look into the possible advantages of LifeWave patches, they frequently find themselves wondering about how to use them, how well they work, and how to take care of them. This chapter explores some of the common questions people have about LifeWave patches and provides helpful tips for resolving typical issues. Grasping these elements can empower individuals to enhance their experience with the patches and make sure they are truly reaping the rewards of their commitment to health and wellness.

1. Frequently Asked Questions About LifeWave Patches

a. How Long to Use the Patch

Many people often wonder how long LifeWave patches should be worn to achieve the best results.

- Recommended Usage: LifeWave patches are generally intended for everyday use. Typically, patches are designed to be worn for 12 hours, after which it's recommended to take a 12-hour break. This cycle helps the body take in the light energy from the patches, while also ensuring that the acupressure points aren't overstimulated.

- Adaptable Usage: Users can modify how long they use the patch based on their personal needs and objectives. Some individuals might opt to wear certain patches for extended periods during times of increased activity, like when preparing for a sports event, or to tackle particular health issues.

- Tune into Your Body: It's important to be in touch with your body and notice how you feel while using the patches. If you feel any discomfort or negative effects, think about wearing it for a shorter time or reaching out to a healthcare professional for advice.

b. Anticipated Timeframes for Observing Outcomes

People often wonder how long it will take to see noticeable results from LifeWave patches. Results can take different amounts of time to appear, depending on various factors like the type of patch used, personal health conditions, and lifestyle choices.

- Personal Differences: Everyone's body reacts uniquely to phototherapy. Things like age, general health, and the particular issue being treated can affect how soon you see results. Some users might feel immediate effects, like a boost in energy or relief from pain, while others may need a few days or even weeks to notice meaningful changes.

- Common Timelines: Although everyone's journey is unique, here are some general timelines for different benefits:
- Energy Boost: Numerous individuals have shared their experiences of feeling more energized just a few days after starting to use the Energy Enhancer patch.
- Pain Relief: Many people find that they feel a noticeable reduction in pain shortly after using the IceWave patch, though those dealing with ongoing pain might need to use it regularly over several weeks to see significant improvement.

- Better Sleep: Many users find that their sleep quality improves within a week of using the Silent Nights patch, though those with ongoing sleep challenges might need a bit more time to see the best results.

- Staying Steady Matters: Regular use of patches is essential for reaching the results you want. Using the patches consistently, together with healthy habits like staying active, drinking enough water, and eating a balanced diet, can really boost your results.

c. Storing and Caring for Patches

Taking good care of LifeWave patches and storing them properly is important for keeping them effective and lasting longer. People frequently wonder about the best ways to manage and store patches properly.

- Storage Conditions: It's best to keep LifeWave patches in a cool, dry spot, away from direct sunlight and heat sources. It's best to keep patches away from extreme temperatures, as doing so can affect how well they work and their overall quality. The best temperature for storage falls between 60°F and 80°F (15°C to 27°C).

- Keep Patches Dry: It's essential to ensure that patches stay moisture-free. Moisture can impact how well the patches stick and might make them less effective. It's best for users to steer clear of using patches in wet settings, like when swimming or taking a shower.

- Handling Precautions: Before applying patches, make sure your hands are clean and dry. Please try not to touch the sticky side of the patches. Oils and dirt from your fingers can impact how well they stick and work.

- Expiration Dates: Each patch is designed to last, usually for about two years from when it was made. It's important for users to take a moment to check the expiration date on the packaging and steer clear of using any expired patches, since they might not work as well.

2. Addressing Common Issues

Even though using LifeWave patches is generally simple, some users might face a few hurdles along the way. Here are some typical worries and helpful suggestions to tackle them in a thoughtful way.

a. Skin Irritation or Allergic Reactions

Some users might notice a bit of skin irritation or have an allergic reaction where the patch is applied. This might happen because of a sensitivity to the adhesive or other ingredients in the patch.

- What to Do: If you experience any irritation, please take off the patch right away and gently wash the area with mild soap and water. Think about using a gentle lotion or aloe vera gel to help soothe your skin. If the irritation continues or gets worse, please reach out to a healthcare professional.

- Patch Placement: Consider placing the patch in another area on your body. People can explore different acupressure points to discover a spot that feels comfortable for them.

b. Patches Not Adhering

Sometimes, people might notice that patches don't stick to the skin as well as they should, which can reduce how well they work.

- Prepare Your Skin: Make sure your skin is clean and dry before applying. Oils, lotions, or sweat can impact how well things stick.

- Explore Various Spots: If a patch isn't adhering well in one place, consider trying it on a different area. Regions with minimal hair or fewer skin folds might offer improved adhesion.

- Use a Skin Barrier: If you have oily skin or tend to sweat a lot, placing a light barrier, like a small piece of medical tape, over the patch can help it stick better.

c. Absence of Outcomes

When users find that the patches aren't delivering the benefits they anticipated, it can be quite disheartening.

- Review Usage Guidelines: Make sure you're using the patches properly and adhering to the suggested guidelines for how long to wear them and where to place them.

- Be Patient: Keep in mind that everyone is different, and it might take a while to see meaningful changes. It's important to use it consistently.

- Incorporate with Daily Habits: To boost the benefits of LifeWave patches, think about weaving in healthy daily habits, like eating well, staying active, and finding ways to manage stress.

d. Talking with Healthcare Providers

If you have any health issues or are on medication, it's a good idea to talk to a healthcare professional before beginning LifeWave patch therapy.

- Medical Guidance: Healthcare providers can provide tailored advice on how to use LifeWave patches alongside other treatments. They can also keep an eye on any changes in symptoms and offer extra support if necessary.

- Addressing Concerns: If you notice any unexpected side effects or have worries about the patches, talking it over with a healthcare provider can guide you in making informed choices about your health and wellness journey.

Getting to know the common questions and helpful troubleshooting tips about LifeWave patches can really improve users' experiences and help them make the most of this innovative phototherapy. By tackling common worries about how long patches last, when to expect results, and how to store and care for them, people can feel more assured in their use of LifeWave patches.

As research progresses and user experiences grow, our grasp of LifeWave patch therapy will deepen, offering individuals valuable resources to improve their health and well-being. If you're looking for relief from pain, a boost in energy, or better sleep, LifeWave patches provide a simple and accessible way to support your overall well-being.

Troubleshooting Common Issues with LifeWave Patches

LifeWave patches aim to provide various health benefits, such as alleviating pain, boosting energy levels, and enhancing sleep quality. Sometimes, users might face challenges that keep them from getting the results they hope for. In this section, we'll take a closer look at some of the challenges that users often face with LifeWave patches, including feelings of ineffectiveness and questions about where to place the patches. This will also offer helpful troubleshooting strategies to enhance the effectiveness of these innovative phototherapy tools.

1. Steps to Take If Patches Aren't Working

Many users often find themselves feeling that LifeWave patches aren't providing the benefits they hoped for. If you happen to be in this situation, take a moment to think about these troubleshooting steps:

a. Take a Moment to Reflect on Your Expectations

Before making any adjustments or changes, it's important to take a moment to rethink your expectations about using LifeWave patches.

- Recognizing Personal Differences: People can react quite differently to the patches due to various factors like their health, age, lifestyle, and the particular issue they are dealing with. Some users might experience benefits right away, while others may need to use it consistently for a longer time to see results.

- Timeline for Results: Generally, individuals may notice some changes within a few days to weeks, influenced by the specific patch being utilized and their personal health objectives. It's important to remember that patience and consistency play a crucial role; the body might need some time to show results.

Make sure to apply it correctly.

Sometimes, challenges with effectiveness can arise from using something in the wrong way.

- Adhere to Application Guidelines: Take a moment to go over the suggested guidelines for using LifeWave patches. Make sure you're positioning them accurately on the right acupressure points to achieve the desired effect. Every patch comes with its own set of guidelines to ensure the best placement.

- Prepare Your Skin: Make sure the spot where you'll place the patch is clean, dry, and free from any oils, lotions, or creams that could interfere with how well it sticks. Taking the time to prepare your skin can really enhance how well the patches stick and work.

c. Assess the Quality of the Patch

Sometimes, how well the patches work can be affected by their quality or condition.

- Check for Damage: Before applying, take a moment to look over the patch for any signs of damage, like tears or old adhesive that may not work well anymore. A damaged patch might not work as well as it should. If a patch seems to be compromised, it's best to throw it away and grab a new one.

- Check Expiration Dates: LifeWave patches have a shelf life, usually lasting about two years from the manufacturing date. It's important to be mindful of expiration dates, as using expired patches can lead to reduced effectiveness. Always take a moment to check before you use them.

d. Take a Moment to Rethink the Type of Patch Used

LifeWave patches each have their own unique functions. If you're not seeing the results you hoped for, take a moment to think about whether the patch you're using truly fits your individual needs.

- Identify Your Goals: Take a moment to reflect on your health aspirations and make sure the patch you choose supports those personal objectives. If you're looking to boost your energy, the Energy Enhancer patch might be a better fit for you compared to those that primarily target pain relief.

- Explore Other Options: If the patch you're using isn't giving you the results you hoped for, think about trying a different LifeWave patch that focuses on your particular concern. If you're seeking pain relief and not experiencing the results you hoped for with one patch, you might want to try the IceWave patch for better management of your discomfort.

e. Integrate with Other Wellness Practices

Using LifeWave patches alongside other wellness practices can enhance their effectiveness.

- Embrace Healthy Lifestyle Choices: To maximize the advantages of LifeWave patches, think about integrating supportive habits into your daily routine, like enjoying a balanced diet, staying active, managing stress effectively, and ensuring you stay well-hydrated. Their influence can greatly affect our overall health and well-being.

- Pay Attention to Your Body: Notice how your body reacts to various wellness practices while using the patch. Recognizing changes or improvements can assist you in spotting patterns and enhancing your health journey.

2. Tweaking Patch Placement for Improved Outcomes

If you're having trouble with how well LifeWave patches are working, trying a different placement might help improve their effectiveness. Here are a few thoughtful approaches to enhance patch placement:

a. Getting to Know Acupressure Points

LifeWave patches function by gently activating particular acupressure points on the body. Grasping these points is essential for making the most of the advantages.

- Explore Important Acupressure Points: Get to know the acupressure points linked to each LifeWave patch. For example, placing the X39 patch near the spine might enhance its regenerative benefits, whereas the IceWave patch is best applied near the area of discomfort.

- Make Use of Resources: Think about using diagrams or guides that show acupressure points along with their related patches. There are plenty of resources online and in LifeWave product literature that can assist you in finding the best placement.

Try out various places.

If you're not seeing the results you hoped for with a patch, it might help to experiment with applying it in different spots.

- Explore Different Body Areas: If a patch isn't giving you the results you hoped for, consider relocating it to other parts of your body. If you're using a patch for pain relief, you may notice improved results by positioning it nearer to the area that's bothering you or trying it on a different side of your body.

- Recognize Sensitive Areas: Certain acupressure points might be more sensitive or impactful for different people. Notice how your body reacts to different positions and make changes as needed.

c. Think About How You Position Your Body and Move

The effectiveness of patches can also be influenced by how you position your body and the way you move.

- Evaluate Your Routine: Think about how your everyday actions might influence how well the patches work. If you're involved in physical activities that require repetitive movements or put strain on certain areas, it could impact how well the patch works to provide relief.

- Resting Position: Try wearing patches in various positions (sitting, standing, lying down) to discover if it affects how well they work. Some users might experience improved results when they are in a relaxed state, while others may find advantages when they are active.

d. Thoughtfully Combine Patches

For individuals facing various health issues, applying multiple patches at the same time can improve their overall effectiveness.

- Layering Patches: Many people discover that using a combination of patches, like pairing an Energy Enhancer patch with an IceWave patch, can create beneficial effects together. Please remember to adhere to the guidelines for patch usage and try to avoid overstimulating any one area.

- Patch Rotation: Think about a strategy for patch rotation where you switch between different patches that address various issues. This method helps the body stay in tune with the patches and makes sure you're taking care of various aspects of your well-being.

By tackling worries about how well the patches work and improving where they are placed, users can greatly improve their experience with LifeWave patches. There are many ways to enhance the benefits of these innovative phototherapy tools, such as reassessing expectations, ensuring proper application, exploring different patch types, or trying out acupressure points.

Everyone's experience with LifeWave patches can be different, and it might take a little while to find what suits you best. By using LifeWave patches correctly, integrating them into your daily life, and being patient, you can truly tap into their full potential on your path to improved health and wellness.

THE END

9bed1582-682c-4182-a139-4718675d9bc5R01